The DARK SIDE of AESTHETICS

HYPERPIGMENTATION, CHEMICAL PEELS, AND COMPLICATIONS

The DARK SIDE of AESTHETICS

HYPERPIGMENTATION, CHEMICAL PEELS, AND COMPLICATIONS

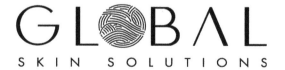

GLOBAL
SKIN SOLUTIONS

GLOBAL SKIN SOLUTIONS PUBLISHING
THE VILLAGES, FLORIDA

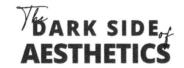

The DARK SIDE of AESTHETICS

HYPERPIGMENTATION, CHEMICAL PEELS, AND COMPLICATIONS

The Villages, Florida
info@pamelaspringer.com

Pamela R. Springer, Publisher / Editorial Director
Yvonne Rose/QualityPress.info, Book Packager

© Copyright 2023 by Pamela R. Springer.
ISBN #: 978-1-0880-2698-4
Library of Congress Control Number: 2023905681

The Dark Side of Aesthetics was my calling to assist aestheticians in reducing the unspeakable facial damage this industry is causing to "skin of color" clients. It is my heartfelt desire to share the knowledge I have to help reduce one of the cosmetic industry's highest liability claims - chemical peel burns.

DEDICATION

This book is dedicated to my mother, father, and brother who are with me in spirit, guiding me to continue my journey as it has been written.

ACKNOWLEDGEMENTS

My heartfelt thanks to my beautiful niece, Keisha, who continues to support me in every aspect of my journey.

A special thanks to my editor and friend, Yvonne Rose, who encourages me to follow my passion and share it with others.

Tina McCaffry, your brilliant mind always knows how to organize my mind, making me think deeper, to give the best of what I know.

Last, but not least, the Grants, Ken & Mary, you have been so supportive since I moved to a new home. You helped me cut through every kind of challenge that came my way. You both are truly special in my life!

To the many aestheticians and medical providers, who have attended my courses, you have validated your commitment to a higher level of knowledge and continued learning. You have demonstrated that you are skilled and experienced to provide the skincare needs of diverse skin tones. Thank you for choosing me to prepare you to be a critical thinker on your educational goals.

CONTENTS

Your face is your billboard. It is the first thing people tend to look at when you walk into a room. Performing advanced services on any skin without the proper knowledge is an accident waiting to happen; therefore, the information in this book has been compiled as a teaching tool to guide you through the proper treatments.

PREFACE

Symone is a beautiful woman of African descent. Her occupation - flight attendant - requires her to maintain and care for her physical appearance. From time to time, I surf the web for ongoing skin care challenges; many of which are frequently seen on Instagram and Tik Tok.

On one such occasion I saw photos of Symone, a skin therapist's client, who had suffered from 2nd degree burns and an acquired fungus infection of her face due to an improper peel treatment. I was troubled by the amount of damage to Symone's skin, and I felt compelled to write this book, *The Dark Side of Aesthetics.*

The severity of 2nd and 3rd degree burns using TCA is astounding, especially for diverse skin tones. These skin tones, rich in melanin, have a higher risk to hyperpigmentation. But because they don't do the proper research about the variables of product usage on diverse skin tones, many skin therapists do more harm than good to their clients. In Symone's case, she stated that there was no skin analysis done when her skin therapist suggested a chemical peel for her dark spots.

A consultation, which includes health issues, family history, allergic reactions, client expectations, etc. is mandatory for gathering information about that client's objective for their initial visit. Next, there should be a skin analysis to ascertain information regarding the skin's barrier and any acute skin condition.

Symone relayed to me that the primary reason for the peel was due to her acne outbreak and the post acne dark spots (hyperpigmentation) on her skin. Since there was no new documentation gathered, it is assumed Symone's barrier was intact due to the previous facials give prior to the TCA chemical peel service. *See case study in Part Two of this book.*

Knowledge is POWER and with it comes MONEY! The next time you have a client or patient on your facial bed, ask yourself, if you would allow a skincare therapist to perform this service on you with the knowledge you have?

INTRODUCTION

The Global market is one of the fastest growing markets in the U.S. for Descendants of Africa, Asians, and Hispanics/Latinos. This growth of ethnic diversity replaces baby boomers as the critical demographic within the U.S. Yet, skincare practitioners are not introduced, in their initial training, to the anatomy and physiology differences of each ethnic group. This lack of knowledge compromises the exploratory phase of a skin analysis and any underlying issues, conclusions or treatment recommendations that may result in a negative outcome.

Skincare practitioners relying on the Fitzpatrick scale have inaccurate indicators when predicting sun sensitivities in an ethnically diverse population. This scale also lacks determining the risk factors of a peel or laser treatment on pigmented skin. A knowledge gap in this area can lead to not only a negative outcome but also place the esthetician and clinic in a potentially harmful legal process of complaints, legal actions and potential loss of the business. Poor outcomes lead to a lack of trust with clients and poor online reviews equal a poor reputation.

Why Is It Happening?

Practitioners, whether they are licensed medical providers or licensed skincare professionals who lack training on the anatomy and physiology of different ethnicities or racial groups. Skin types and common skin conditions manifest differently in a white or light skin vs. a melanin rich skin.

The following chapters cover how to:

- achieve a comprehensive overview of the parameters for the skin's exploratory phase.

- use a skin classification system that maximizes the safety professionals should use when working with ethnically challenged skins.

- provide a systematic level of pre-treatment prior to a chemical peel application.

- determine skin conditions' primary and secondary cause.

- choose a chemical peeling agent best suited for the determined epidermal or dermal level.

- manage the complications of a peel when used on light and dark skins.

To be a skincare expert in today's changing landscape, you must understand Global skin types. In the United States, the proportion of the population with diverse skin tones, which includes those of Asian, South Asian, Hispanic, Mediterranean, Middle Eastern, and African descents, is increasing.

It is estimated that 30% of all U.S. cosmetic skin care clients are multi-ethnic skin types. The demand for multi-ethnic skin treatment is expected to soar. Understanding the intricacies of each ethnic group's common skin conditions and the challenge of limiting risk factors, such as post inflammatory hyperpigmentations, is essential or crucial to today's skincare professional.

If you're feeling that you currently do not see these clients in your practice today, think again! Italian and Lebanese are ethnic, no matter how light their skin tone may appear. Not educating yourself on this growing untapped market, will be a missed opportunity to build your business and your reputation.

As we move forward into the 21st century, the ethnic consumer will be an important part of the skin care industry. The U.S. Census Bureau reports by 2050, half of the U.S. population will be people of color, replacing baby boomers as the critical growth demographic. In my opinion, more than 50% of the U.S. population is ethnic. Racial blending has now surpassed Hispanics as the fastest growing demographic group.

Although the skin care industry is still lagging in providing distinctive products and treatments, The Nielsen Company predicts there will be significant growth in this market in the near future. Recently there has been a significant amount of media coverage on products that diminish dark spots, discoloration, and uneven skin tones. Whereas, previously, the concerns were fine lines and wrinkles observed mostly in European skin. Women and men of certain ethnic descents - Middle Eastern, Hispanic, Asian or Descendants of Africa skins need products and services that address their unique skin-related challenges.

Just Look at Me - My Personal Experience!

I would like to first start with my experience when seeking services from a licensed skincare professional. The first step should be a consultation. Since I am a woman of color, during this consultation it should be obvious that my skin color will play an important part in how my skin functions. Getting to know the dynamics of my skin to include the physiological makeup of a "mixed race" skin is important.

So, you ask, *why?* My ancestral makeup or genetic coding includes three different lineages – genetics from the motherland, Africa, as well as Native American, and European descendants. My caramel-colored skin is the result of these different races. With that said, the blending of these races will play a crucial part on how my skin reacts. Also, I may be more prone to certain conditions due to this blending.

With so many people seeking information from a genealogy company, they are discovering their mixed ancestral make up. With this blending of races, many individuals are misdiagnosed by skincare professionals because practitioners were never exposed, in their initial training, to other skin tones except those of a Nordic skin type. The Fitzpatrick scale is used frequently to classify a client's or a patient's phototype. This will only reveal how the skin responds to ultraviolet radiation (UVR) or its tanning ability.

It is important to determine the risk factor of blended skins in order to understand the response when using a chemical peel or laser. A complete overview of various skin classification scales is outlined in Chapter 3.

So, let's start at the very beginning...

PART ONE

A COMPREHENSIVE OVERVIEW

CHAPTER 1

CONSULTATION

W hen a client comes into a skin care salon seeking the services of an aesthetician, there is a plan of action that skin therapists should follow. The following shows the appropriate steps for the preparation of a client's course of treatments.

Achieving a comprehensive overview of the parameters for skin's exploratory consultation.

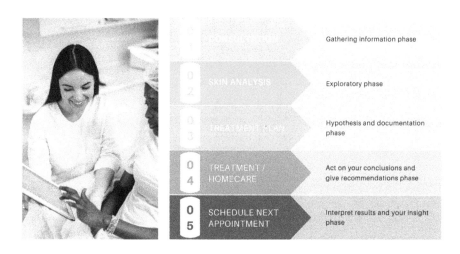

CONSULTATION:

It begins with using a form to gather information that will be vital to the client's well-being.

Confidential Skin Care Evaluation

Please answer the following questions so that your Skin Care Professional may have a better understanding of your general health and life style. This will enable us to accurately analyze and assess your skin care needs.

Name _____ Date _____

Address _____

City _____ State _____ Zip _____

Email _____ Home Phone _____

Date of Birth _____ Cell Phone _____

Receive our Newsletter ❑ Yes ❑ No   Receive Text Messages   ❑ Yes   ❑ No

Emergency Contact Name _____ Phone _____

1. What is the reason for your visit today?

2. What special areas of concern do you have?

❑ Acne scarring	❑ Pigmentation	❑ Age spots
❑ Acne	❑ Sun damage	❑ Fine Lines and wrinkles
❑ Scars or Keloids	❑ Stretch Marks	❑ Ingrown Hairs

3. Have you ever had

❑ Microdermabrasion	❑ LED	❑ Enzyme treatments
❑ Cosmetic surgery	❑ Laser Hair Removal	❑ Body treatments
❑ Cosmetic fillers	❑ Electrolysis in the past 14 days	❑ Chemical peels ____ Percentage?
❑ Botox®?	❑ Dermatitis	❑ Home care with acids
❑ Restylane®	❑ Keloid scarring	❑ Permanent Cosmetics
❑Collagen Injections	❑ At home microdermabrasion	

Comments:

4. Have you seen a Dermatologist in the past Year? ❑ Yes   ❑ No

   Name of dermatologist _____ Reason for visit _____

5. Are you presently under the care of a physician? ❑ Yes   ❑ No   If yes, explain

ALLERGIES/REACTIONS

6. Do you have or ever had a reaction/allergy to

❑ Metals	❑ Chemical or natural peels?	❑ Food
❑ Fragrance	❑ Cosmetics	❑ Airborne particles
❑ Aspirin or Salicylates	❑ Ingredients in cosmetics.	❑ Herbs or flowers

FOR MEN

Do you experience breakouts?   ❑ Yes ❑ No
Do you have ingrown hair?   ❑ Yes ❑ No

FOR WOMEN

Are you on birth control?   ❑ Yes ❑ No
Do you take hormone replacement?   ❑ Yes ❑ No
Are you pregnant?   ❑ Yes ❑ No

The following are a few pertinent questions to add to an intake form.

- Name, address, email address and phone number for emergency purposes.

- Date of birth

  - Knowing a date of birth assists in comparing the condition of the skin with the chronological aging of the client.

- What is the reason for your visit today?

  - This allows you to know exactly what they are expecting to receive.

- What area of concerns do you have?

  - Pointing out what bothers them about their skin gives you a heads up on what to address first.

- Add a line asking for their particular concern or concerns that they would like you to address.

  - This question is probably the most important question that a client will answer. It will open the lines of communication between you and the client.

  - What you might find important to address in the client's skin may not be what the client sees as a problem.

  - Again, this opens the lines of communication. At this point, you can explain to the client the different types of treatments offered.

- o Have a conversation on the understanding that some skin conditions may require more than one treatment to achieve the results desired. And the results cannot be guaranteed due to an individual skin type or skin condition.

- Have you seen a dermatologist?
  - o If your client has seen a dermatologist, receiving the name of the dermatologist will allow you to contact them if you have any questions.
  - o It also will let you know they may be having a treatment that is out of your scope of practice, or it gives an indication that the client is on a prescription medication.

- Ask, what are their expectations of the treatment today and document their answer.
  - o Again, this opens the lines of communication. At this point, you can explain to the client the different types of treatments offered.

- Occupation
  - o An occupation will help rule out any type of occupational hazard to the skin – Example – working in a greasy kitchen.
    - ▪ The greasy environment may be the cause of blackheads, whiteheads or acne breakouts seen on the client's skin.

- Chemical Peels – (last service and how often)
    - Knowing how often the client is receiving AHA or BHA Retinols, and Retin A. These ingredients in their home care regimen will determine if it may be the cause of skin sensitivity.

- Tanning beds
    - If they use tanning beds, educate the client on what the risk factors are of UVA rays being emitted from this equipment.
    - If the answer is yes, ask the client when was the last time they were used.
    - This activity will have to cease if the treatment plan will include the use of a PRO peel application.

- Genetic coding (DNA):

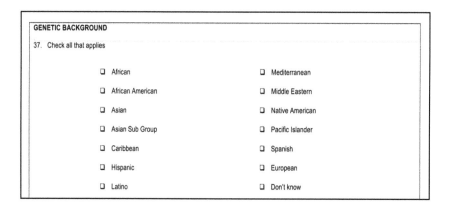

GENETIC BACKGROUND

37. Check all that applies

☐ African	☐ Mediterranean
☐ African American	☐ Middle Eastern
☐ Asian	☐ Native American
☐ Asian Sub Group	☐ Pacific Islander
☐ Caribbean	☐ Spanish
☐ Hispanic	☐ European
☐ Latino	☐ Don't know

- Medical History

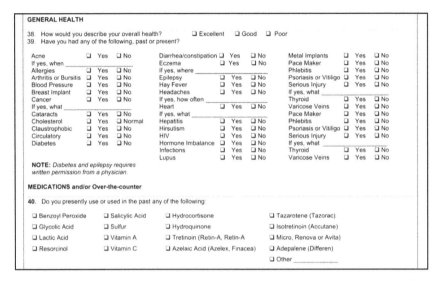

o Having a full medical history is important. Knowing if your client is under the care of a physician will let you know if certain treatments should be administered. If you are not sure if a treatment can be administered, ask the client to get approval from their physician on the physician's letterhead. This document should be saved or scanned in a file to show documentation if a service becomes a legal action suit.

o Have the client list all the medications and vitamins they are currently taking.

  ▪ Sometimes medication can be the cause of a skin's condition. A list of all medication taken will give you a better assessment of the client condition.

- This is when you should purchase a PDR – Physician's Desk Reference. – This book will give you the generic and the trademark drug names of all medications. You can purchase on Amazon as a paperback. It will also tell you if you can or cannot administer a chemical peel while on a particular drug.

- Allergies

  - There are allergies that will restrict certain PRO treatments, i.e., if a client is allergic to aspirin, salicylic should not be used since salicylic is an aspirin compound.

  - Allergies to skin care products or ingredients must be documented in the client's file notes. Most clients know what they have a reaction to and how certain ingredients will affect them. If they are not sure of a reaction, before applying a chemical peel do a patch test 24 to 48 hours before the the peel service on the side of the client's neck. Also apply the chemical along the jawline or behind the ear. Call or have the client report the results within 24 to 48 hours after an application.

- Include a question regarding the client taking any type of hormone therapy or if they are on birth control pills.

  - If so, this may explain any acne breakouts or melasma.

- o Retin-A should be addressed if in the past 3 months. If the client checks, yes, ask how often and at what percentage.

  - Retin-A is an exfoliant that may leave the skin red and/or sensitive. It is important to inform the client they may have to discontinue their Retin-A if a peel will be administered in the future. Be sure to highlight the strength and how often the drug is used.

- o Another Vitamin A derivative is isotretinoin.

  - This drug is potent. It is prescribed for cystic acne. The client follows up with their doctor monthly.

  - Females must be on birth control pills to insure they do not get pregnant.

  - The negative side effect is that it not only dries up the sebum within the sebaceous glands, but also the whole body is affected.

  - Some clients will use eye drops to keep their eyes wet.

  - This drug causes the skin to constantly shed in a rapid timeframe. For this main reason you do not want to do any type of exfoliation, waxing, or peels.

- The PRO treatment performed should be the use of enzymes and hydrating products with an oil-based moisturizer to lock the moisture into the skin layers.

o Record any other health problems, past or present.

- Diabetes, heart, hepatitis, thyroid conditions, cancer, cyst, hormonal, acne high blood pressure.

- Many of these health issues will require omission of certain treatments and the use of certain equipment used in treatments. This information should be documented, highlighted, and saved in the client notes that can be reviewed each time the client comes in for a service.

- Skin Conditions

---

1. What is the reason for your visit today?

2. What special areas of concern do you have?

❏ Acne scarring	❏ Pigmentation	❏ Age spots
❏ Acne	❏ Sun damage	❏ Fine Lines and wrinkles
❏ Scars or Keloids	❏ Stretch Marks	❏ Ingrown Hairs

3. Have you ever had

❏ Microdermabrasion	❏ LED	❏ Enzyme treatments
❏ Cosmetic surgery	❏ Laser Hair Removal	❏ Body treatments
❏ Cosmetic fillers	❏ Electrolysis in the past 14 days	❏ Chemical peels ____ Percentage?
❏ Botox®?	❏ Dermatitis	❏ Home care with acids
❏ Restylane®	❏ Keloid scarring	❏ Permanent Cosmetics
❏ Collagen Injections	❏ At home microdermabrasion	

Comments:

4. Have you seen a Dermatologist in the past Year? ❏ Yes ❏ No

Name of dermatologist _____ Reason for visit _____

5. Are you presently under the care of a physician? ❏ Yes ❏ No If yes, explain

o   If acne prone is checked, ask if they consume a lot of cheese or milk.

- Dairy cows are treated with artificial hormones that affect their milk supply. Researchers suggest that those hormones may throw your hormones off balance when milk products are consumed. This is a known trigger for acne.

- Another theory is that the growth hormones already in milk naturally aggravate acne, no matter what.

- A third theory is that milk products, when combined with the high levels of refined foods and processed sugars in the Western diet, disrupt insulin levels and make skin more prone to acne.

o   Oral herpes, fever blisters or cold sores?

- If any type of chemical peel is going to be recommended, they need to see a physician for the appropriate treatment for at least one week prior to the peeling treatment. Herpes simplex virus is activated with excessive exfoliation and stimulation to the skin.

- Surgeries
  - Ask if they've had any plastic surgery or laser treatment in the past three months.
    - If so, it is recommended that the client or patient check with their physician prior to any skin care or body care treatments.
- Pregnancy
  - It is important to know if the client or patient is pregnant. If pregnant, document how many months.
  - Your inquiry to these questions is not to be nosy, but to be aware of what you can and cannot do in treatments.
  - Check with the client's physician prior to any skincare or body care treatments if it is before three months.
    - A pregnant women's skin is more sensitive because the body and skin are going through changes. Chemical peels are not recommended if a client is pregnant.
- Family History
  - List skin conditions that may be inherited, i.e., acne, melasma, keloids, etc.
    - A client inherits half of their genetic profile from each parent. Along with the genetic

information that determines your appearance, you also inherit genes that might cause or increase your risk of certain medical or skin conditions. A family medical history can reveal the history of disorders in their family, which can help you identify the overall outcome of treatment modalities.

▪ Because many individuals are mixed with other races, ask the client to check off all that applies to their genetic makeup. This will give you an idea of certain skin conditions that may be prevalent in a certain race that may appear on the skin of someone who would not normally have these skin conditions.

- For example – rosacea. In our initial training, rosacea was stated as a condition only prevalent in northern European skins – such as Irish, German, etc. Rosacea is seen in Asians, African Americans, and Hispanics/Latinos/Spanish skins. My theory is that if you are mixed with northern European race, you may be prone to rosacea.

- Have a commitment clause.

  o This allows the practitioner to receive a commitment to services recommended.

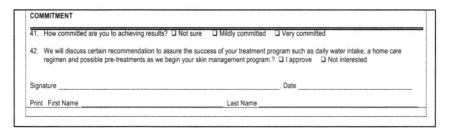

- The client signs the intake form and dates it on the day of the consultation.

- Each week, the client should sign a waiver stating that all the information provided was true and correct to the best of their knowledge. The client signs this waiver each time they come in. For anyone filing a liability claim, this is documentation that can be used as a form of consent.

WAIVER

I acknowledge that all the information provided by me is true and correct to the best of my knowledge.

I understand that some skin conditions may require more than one treatment to achieve the results desired. Results cannot be guaranteed due to individual skin type and skin condition.

Signature: _____

I understand I need to sign this waiver prior to every treatment provided with ANY changes pertaining to the above questionnaire noted.

Treatment:
Client Signature _____ Date: _____

Treatment:

Client Signature _____ Date: _____

Treatment:

Client Signature _____ Date: _____

Treatment:

Client Signature _____ Date: _____

Treatment:

Client Signature _____ Date: _____

Treatment:

Client Signature _____ Date: _____

Treatment:

Client Signature _____ Date: _____

Treatment:

Client Signature _____ Date: _____

CHAPTER 2

SKIN ANALYSIS

The goal of skin analysis is to collect the information you need to improve the client's appearance. The more you know, the better equipped you are to make recommendations.

A thorough examination of the skin using the proper equipment is necessary to develop a treatment plan. Before embarking on a treatment plan, one must have a thorough knowledge of the skin's anatomy. This visual assessment should be conducted whenever the client comes in for a treatment. These continued visual assessments record the client's progress and if there is a need to change the treatment plan's documentation.

- The use of the following visual diagnostic tools will ascertain the condition of the skin. If a previous treatment has been administered, doing a visual assessment using these tools will dictate the skin's need to repeat the previous treatment or to administer a more advanced protocol.

- It is important to have the tools for accuracy of the analysis of the skin.

    o It is important to touch skin.

- Examining the skin by touch allows you to feel the texture, the temperature, how oily or dry. Gently pinch the skin to feel the thickness or thinness of the skin. Visually, look for any redness, rashes, clogged pores. Look for signs of a skin condition – hyperpigmentation, acne, eczema, etc.

o Magnifying lamp

- Confirms the manual analysis. It gives a closer view of the skin's surface.

- Look for pore size, clogged pores, congestion, sun damage, freckles, and any abnormalities – for instance – irregular-looking lesions suggesting skin cancer.

o Moisture Checker

- Measures water content in the skin.

- Checks the moisture level before and after applying a product.

o Ultra-violet lamp

- A Wood's Lamp, Skin Scanner, or ultraviolet light camera.

- These devices confirm skin irregularities you can't see with the naked eye.

- Woods Lamp-emits ultraviolet light at a wavelength of 320-400nm.

- Epidermis is visible.

- Dermis not visible - abnormalities are not visible.

- Defines dry and oily areas.

- Thickness of skin detected.

- Confirms deeper damage and pigmentation disorders (hyper- or hypopigmentation.

- Can show any skin fungus.

- Reveals the healthy skin areas.

- When performing chemical peels, a Woods lamp is a very useful guide to help with a peeling solution. The purpose is to note an even application of the product to all areas. Woods lamps also help with assessing the protective value of sunscreens and barrier creams. The use of this lamp gives the aesthetician the opportunity to recommend and sell the correct treatment and retail products to their clients.

- An interactive tool that allows your client to be involved. They quickly see their own hidden skin conditions. Using a Skin Scanner makes skin analysis simple, accurate and fun! Using the color chart, it easily identifies sun damage, dehydration, oily or dry skin. The different conditions show up as various colors.

- A great maintenance tool for a client to see before and after results at the end of a service. This will continue to be an ideal way of monitoring a client's progress throughout a series of skin care treatments.

Woods Lamp Chart

Color	Indications
Blue/White	Normal, Healthy skin
White Spots	Horny layer buildup
Purple Florescent	Thin, Dehydrated
Light Violet	Dry
Bright Florescent	Hydrated, dewy
Orange/Coral	Oily areas & comedones
Brown	Hyper-pigmentation (freckles & dark spots)

Let's Recap!

- Always keep in mind the realistic goals and the client's goals and expectations.

- Establish your goals!

- Do not perform any service that is outside your comfort level or scope of practice.

- Perform an initial treatment using enzymes to see how the skin responds.

- Determine the skin's immediate facial treatment needs.

Complete the skin analysis form

Global Skin Solutions

SKIN ANALYSIS   Client Name _____   Date _____

VASCULAR SYSTEM

Normal	❏	Erythema	❏
Telangiectasia	❏	Angioma	❏

LIPIDIC SYSTEM

Sebaceous secretions: normal ❏ hypersecretions (greasy or oily) ❏ hyposecretions (alipic or dry) ❏
seborrheic ❏ combination ❏ asphyxic ❏ comedonal ❏ acneic ❏

Macules	❏	Pustules	❏
Nodules	❏	Nodules	❏
Papules	❏	Vesicles	❏
Outbreaks: rare ❏	intermittent ❏	consistent ❏	numerous ❏

EPIDERMIC HYDRIC SYSTEM

		SENSITIVITY AND REACTIVITY	
Normal Hydration	❏	Normal	❏
Dehydration:		Reactive	❏
Superficial	❏	Hyper-reactive	❏
Deep	❏	Rosacea	❏
Wrinkles	❏		
Fine lines	❏		
Furrows	❏		

TEXTURE

Skin Texture:	fine (few pores or not noticeable)	❏
	some pores (somewhat noticeable)	❏
	noticeable pores	❏
Skin Thickness	fine	❏
	normal (medium)	❏
	thick	❏

SKIN TONE / COMPLEXION

SKIN TONE		COMPLEXION			
Firm	❏	Normal	❏	Bilious	❏
Slightly loose	❏	Redness	❏	Clear	❏
Flaccid	❏	Dull	❏	Golden	❏
Double chin	❏	Sallow	❏	Pinkish	❏
Eyelid ptosis	❏	Pale	❏		

PIGMENTATION

Hyperchromias: freckles ❏ lentigos ❏ nevus ❏ age spots ❏ melasma ❏

EYE CONTOUR ANALYSIS

Aqueous pockets	❏	Wrinkles	❏
Lipidic pockets (fat)	❏	Circulatory circles	❏
Xanthomas	❏	Pigmentary circles	❏
Milia	❏	Eyelid edema	❏
Fine lines	❏		

COMMENTS
_____
_____

A completed form will help to establish:

- Skin type – primary cause.

    o Normal to dry-dehydrated, moisture/dry, oily/dry.

    o Normal to oily-enlarged pores, congested, comedones, whiteheads, and acne.

- Skin conditions – secondary cause

    o Sensitive, pregnancy mask (chloasma), psoriasis, eczema, rosacea, facial hair, dark circles, environmentally damaged, traumatized skin, and adult acne.

CHAPTER 3

SKIN CLASSIFICATIONS

The use of a skin classification will maximize the safety that professionals should use when working with ethnically challenged skin.

It is important to understand the ancestral makeup or genetics of a client or patient. To do this, there are various skin classification scales to assist in providing information on many of the risk factors that those with pigmented skin may have from advanced treatments, including chemical peel agents and laser treatments.

We learned to use the Fitzpatrick Scale in our initial training. Unfortunately, Fitzpatrick VI states that this phototype does not burn, when indeed it does. Granted, this phototype would have to stay in the sun much longer, than say, a Fitzpatrick I or II phototype.

My research unveiled the Lancer ethnicity scale, which noted risk factors using a numeric scale.

Most recently, I discovered the Genetico-Racial Skin Classification, which not only outlined risk factors but also gives an in-depth description of the facial features along with the skin's thickness.

Let's start with one of the earlier classifications, which more or less detects the aging process of a Nordic skin type.

Glogau's Classifications of Photoaging Groups

- **Mild aging**: ages 28 – 35. Little wrinkling or scarring. No keratosis. Requires no makeup.

- **Moderate aging**: ages 35 – 50. Early wrinkling, mild scarring. Sallow color with early actinic keratosis. Requires little makeup.

- **Advanced aging**: ages 50 – 65 Persistent wrinkling or moderate acne scarring. Discoloration with telangiectasia and actinic keratosis. Wears makeup always.

- **Severe aging**: ages 60 – 75 Wrinkling, photoaging, gravitational, and dynamic, actinic keratosis with or without skin cancer or severe acne scars. Wears make-up with poor coverage.

Fitzpatrick Scale

The Fitzpatrick Scale offers a useful method of classifying a patient's skin phototype. This scale does little to predict the skin's response to trauma from certain procedures, such as chemical peels, laser treatments or surgeries. This system is potentially misleading, as all skin types to include Fitzpatrick types V and VI are susceptible to some element of burning from UV radiation. The Fitzpatrick phototype scale, which is based on the propensity of an individual to burn and tan, initially had only four classifications; types V and

VI were subsequently added for Asian Indians and African aboriginal people, respectively.

A skin classification should also predict how the skin reacts to various modalities, such as chemical peels and laser treatments. It should also point out the possible complications to these treatments.

The other important piece of information is to know that one's ancestral makeup is important for the possibility of being prone to certain skin conditions, i.e., rosacea. Rosacea is mostly associated with people from Northern Europe (Nordic skin) or whose ancestral make up is mixed with Northern European ancestry.

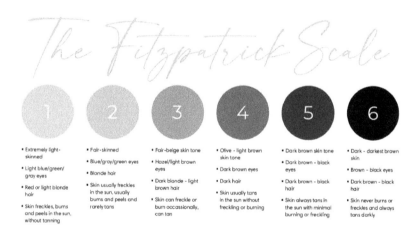

The Fitzpatrick Scale

1	2	3	4	5	6
• Extremely light-skinned	• Fair-skinned	• Fair-beige skin tone	• Olive - light brown skin tone	• Dark brown skin tone	• Dark - darkest brown skin
• Light blue/green/gray eyes	• Blue/gray/green eyes	• Hazel/light brown eyes	• Dark brown eyes	• Dark brown - black eyes	• Brown - black eyes
• Red or light blonde hair	• Blonde hair	• Dark blonde - light brown hair	• Dark hair	• Dark brown - black hair	• Dark brown - black hair
• Skin freckles, burns and peels in the sun, without tanning	• Skin usually freckles in the sun, usually burns and peels and rarely tans	• Skin can freckle or burn occassionally, can tan	• Skin usually tans in the sun without freckling or burning	• Skin always tans in the sun with minimal burning or freckling	• Skin never burns or freckles and always tans darkly

Lancer Ethnicity Scale

The Lancer Ethnicity Scale includes the Fitzpatrick Scale to determine risk factor for chemical peels and lasers. The scale breakdown is for European skins and those with minimally to melanin-rich pigmented skins from various geographical locations.

Lancer Ethnicity Scale

Appropriate and effective treatments can't always be calculated by a patient's skin type by just looking. The critical missing component is the patient's ethnic background.

LES works by calculating healing efficacy and risk factors based on the ethnic backgrounds of all four grandparents combined. Risk factors include keloids, discoloration, scar atrophy, enlarged pore size and prolonged healing. The higher the LES indicator is, the greater likelihood for healing difficulties.

- To calculate your client's skin on the Lancer Ethnicity Scale, find the LES Skin type numbers for each of their grandparents.
- Add the numbers together and divide this total by four.

Keeping in mind that no chemical peeling, laser or surgery procedure is risk free. The lower your LES Skin Type, the better your skin healing should be after a chemical exfoliation, laser, cosmetic or traditional surgery and the less risk there is of scarring, keloids, erythema, discoloration and uneven pigmentation.

LANCER ETHNICITY SCALE (LES)

ANCESTRAL BACKGROUND	LES	Risk Factors
Celtic (Ireland, Scotland, Wales), Nordic (Denmark, Finland, Iceland, Norway, Sweden)	Skin Type 1	Very Low Risk
Central/Eastern European (Austria, Czech Republic) Hungary, Poland, Croatia, Ukraine, Latvia)	Skin Type 2	Low Risk
Ashkenazy Jewish, Mediterranean Countries (Spain, Portugal, Italy, Greece)	Skin Type 3	Moderate Risk
Asian (Chinese, Korean, Thai, Vietnamese, Polynesian) Sephardic Jewish (Spanish & Portuguese)	Skin Type 4	Significant Risk
African, African American	Skin Type 5	Considerable Risk

Fitzpatrick Phototype

Skin Type I - Never tans, always burns
(extremely fair skin, blonde hair, blue/ green eyes)
Skin Type II - Occasionally tans, usually burns
(fair skin, sandy to brown hair, green/brown eyes)
Skin Type III - Often tans, sometimes burns
(medium skin, brown hair, brown eyes)
Skin Type IV - Always tans, never burns
(olive skin, brown/black hair, dark brown/black eyes)
Skin Type V - Never burns
(dark brown skin, black hair, black eyes)
Skin Type VI - Never burns
(black skin, black hair, black eyes)

There are many other scales, but the following Genetico-Racial Classification scale is the latest.

THE GENETICO-RACIAL CLASSIFICATION

The Genetico-Racial Classification scale encompasses skin color; facial features of the descendants of Africa, Asia, and Europe; and the side effects or complications as it pertains to each risk factor that may occur.

The scale divides the descendants of the three ancient continents into six genetico-racial subtypes; describes the incremental changes in skin color; skin thickness, and facial characteristic.

Across Europe and Africa

- The Nordics: individuals *originating* from northern Europe (e.g., Scandinavian, Irish or Scottish roots).

- The Europeans: individuals *originating* from mid-Europe (e.g., German, English, northern Spanish, northern Italian, Polish or French roots).

- The Mediterraneans: individuals *originating* from southern Europe, most northern Africa and western middle Asia (e.g., southern Italian, southern Spanish, Portuguese, Greek, Lebanese or Iranian roots).

- The Indo-Pakistanis: individuals *originating* from upper-middle Africa, western lower Asia (e.g., Pakistani, Thai, Indian, Egyptian or Saudi roots).

- The Africans: individuals *originating* from middle and lower Africa (e.g., Sudanese, Ethiopian or South African roots).

Across Central and Eastern Asia

- The Asians: individuals *originating* from central and eastern Asia (e.g., Korean, Chinese, Japanese or Philippino roots).

Summary of the characteristics and responses of the different genetico-racial categories

Racial category	Original geographical habitat	Characteristics of skin and facial features	Side effects/complications	Rating as candidate
Nordics (e.g.: Swedish, Irish)	Northern Europe	Color: white to very white Skin: thin Features: fine (small noses, thin lips, etc.)	• Erythema +++ • Telangiectasia + • Scarring	• Very good
Europeans (e.g.: French, English)	Mid-Europe	Color: white or light tan Skin: average thickness Features: average size	Low incidence	• Excellent
Mediterranean (e.g.: Spanish, Greek)	Southern Europe, most northern Africa, western Asia	Color: medium tan Skin: slightly thick Features: slightly coarse	• Erythema + to ++ • Hyperpigmentation + to ++	• Very good
Indo-Pakistanis (e.g.: Pakistani, Thai)	Northern Africa, southern Asia	Color: deep tan to dark brown Skin: thick Features: moderate to coarse	• Hyperpigmentation +++ • Hypopigmentation +	• Good for medium peels • Passable for deep peels or light laser resurfacing

Skin Classifications

Racial category	Original geographical habitat	Characteristics of skin and facial features	Side effects/complications	Rating as candidate
Africans (e.g.: Black American, Sudanese)	Middle and lower Africa	Color: black to deep black Skin: thick to very thick Features: slightly coarse to very coarse	• Hyperpigmentation +++ • Hypopigmentation ++	• Passable for light to medium peels • Poor for deep peels or laser resurfacing
Asians (e.g.: Japanese, Korean)	Central Asia, eastern Asia	A separate classification Color: varies from light to medium to dark Skin: thick to very thick Features: coarse to very coarse	• Hyperpigmentation +++ • Erythema ++, turning to hyperpigmentation	• Good
Asians (e.g.: Japanese, Korean)	Central Asia, eastern Asia	A separate classification Color: varies from light to medium to dark Skin: thick to very thick Features: coarse to very coarse	• Hyperpigmentation +++ • Erythema ++, turning to hyperpigmentation	• Good

A1, A2 – Examples of patients with Nordic roots: pale white thin skin, fine features.

B1, B2 – Examples of patients with European roots: white or slightly tanned skin, medium features.

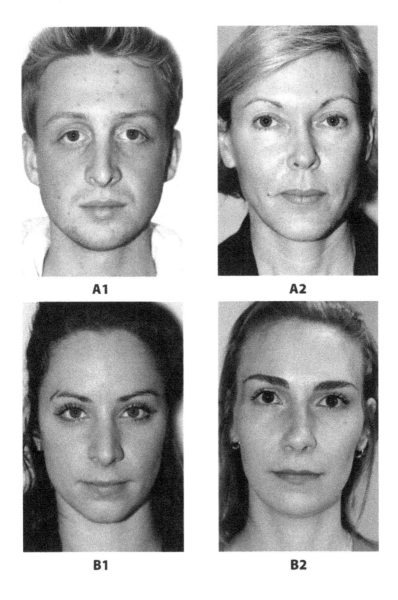

A1

A2

B1

B2

C1, C2 – Examples of patients with Mediterranean roots: darker tanned skin, mildly coarse features.

D1, D2 – Examples of patients with Indo-Pakistani roots: medium to deep brown thick skin, moderately coarse features.

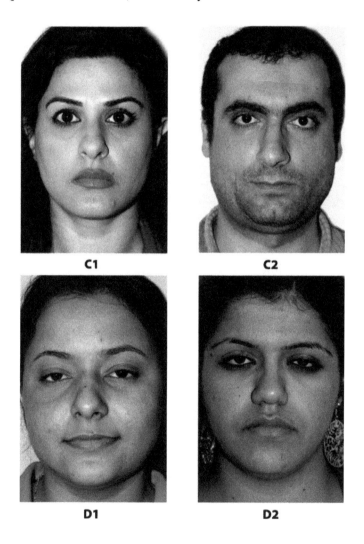

C1   C2

D1   D2

E1, E2 – Examples of patients with African roots: black thick skin, very coarse features.

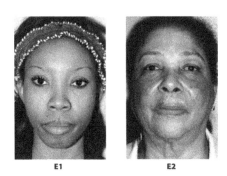

Examples of patients with Asian roots – Northern Asian (F1): white or mildly tanned skin, mildly coarse features; Central Asian (F2): medium tanned skin, moderately coarse features; Southern Asian (F3): medium to dark brown skin, coarse features.

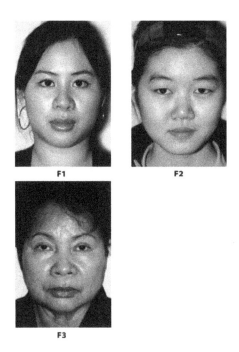

Origins versus country of residence

In all instances, patients should be classified according to their 'country of origin' rather than their 'country of residence.' In other words, the skin of an African American is classified as 'African' even if he/she lives in Alaska. Likewise, the skin of a South African citizen, who is white with an Irish descent, is still classified as 'Nordic'.

CHAPTER 4

TREATMENT PLAN

WHERE TO BEGIN!

Barrier Function

Corneotherapy is a newer field of skin treatment within the fields of dermatology and aesthetics. It is all about repairing, restoring, and regenerating the skin barrier, while aiming for long-term stabilization of the skin barrier.

What is corneotherapy? It was not until the 1960s that dermatologist and co-inventor of Retin-A, Dr. Albert Kligman, and his partners discovered that the stratum corneum is actually alive, and not a layer of dead cells waiting to shed. This finding gave way to what is known today as corneotherapy. Corneotherapy centers on corneobiology – an anatomy, physiology, and biology of the stratum corneum-based science.

A key principle of corneotherapy is to always keep the epidermis intact, with the therapeutic actions working from the outer layers of the epidermis inward. This approach of retaining the integrity of the epidermis ensures the skin's defense and immune systems are not stimulated unnecessarily.

With the current knowledge, we now know that it is not necessarily the deeper skin layers that have to be stimulated and supported with active agents, but rather the uppermost skin layer (Stratum Corneum) that is known as the horny layer now offers interesting areas for new thinking and concepts.

This is why it is important to establish the barrier's (acid mantle) state of health and the primary and secondary causes of the skin condition(s) through the analysis pathway model. A compromised barrier shows the skin type to be dry, oily, sensitive or a combination of dry and oily.

Once you determine the skin type, it is important to determine the primary cause of the issue. Is it dry because the client is -

- Taking medication

  o Skin will continue to be dry as long as the client is taking medication. Keeping the skin hydrated will be the primary fix. Therefore, the client will have home care, water-based products with an occlusive moisturizer for both home care management products as well as hydrating PRO treatments.

- Moved or just moved to a dry climate.

  o Normally, it may take up to 2 years for the skin to acclimate to the new climate.

- Using skin care products that are stripping the barrier's natural oils.

- o Removing harsh ingredients and implementing hydrating home care management products as well as hydrating PRO treatment modalities will reduce skin sensitivity and repair the compromised barrier.

Dry skin treatment guidelines are as follows:

- Begin all treatments with an enzyme as the exfoliant. If the goal is to perform advanced exfoliating (chemical peels, microdermabrasion, etc.), slowly introduce these services after the barrier function has been restored. Remember these services remove the barrier and it will have to be, again, restored.

- Clients must comply with the home care preparation. If they are not following your recommendation, continue with the in-clinic enzyme as an exfoliant.

It is important that time is allowed to rebuild the skin at a gradual pace. This will take two to three weeks. Once the barrier is intact, you can address the skin condition.

Products should include a cleanser, toner, serum, moisturizer, and sun block. If a client is not able to purchase all the products recommended, choose a product like a serum (hyaluronic) that has active ingredients and any additional product(s) the client is missing from their skin regimen.

Dry Skins: Products should contain both a humectant as well as oil-based moisturizer ingredients to assist in "locking" moisture into the layers of the skin.

Oily Skins: Products should be of a water-based formula. Adding hydration to the skin helps to reduce the sebaceous gland activity.

Until the acid mantle is repaired, refrain from the use of chemical peeling agents.

CHAPTER 5

HOME CARE

HOME CARE MANAGEMENT PROGRAM

- Suggest home care products.

- Follow-up appointment (weekly, bi-monthly, or monthly)

- Following up with client 24-48 hours after an initial visit

- Set goals and document on treatment plan.

Issues clients have:

- Lasers and Retinols

  Laser and retinol treated skin should be considered sensitive skin.

- Face lifts

  Recent face-lift clients should always be treated cautiously, even while waxing. Complete healing from plastic surgery takes six to nine months.

- Photo-rejuvenation

  Pigmentation that has not responded to lightening products after a minimum of six months of continual use can be reevaluated and referred to the dermatologist or plastic surgeon for photo-rejuvenation with appropriate lasers. No photo facial or IPL or Thermolysis. During the series of treatments, it is not recommended to do aggressive treatments or waxing. It may be useful to continue using pigment lightening gel and AHAs. NO microdermabrasion treatments can be useful to reduce flakiness. After photo-rejuvenation treatments, anti-aging and antioxidant creams are often more effective.

- Previous existing conditions

  Patients with previous existing conditions such as eczema, psoriasis, and rosacea need to be worked with on an individual basis. Begin cautiously using sensitive products, less heat/steam and less physical massage with more focus on pressure point and lymphatic drainage type massage. Because these conditions are easily aggravated by stress, it is suggested that they maintain doctor care for these conditions.

- Menopause, Stress skin or Rosacea

  Menopause and stress skin may react best with a combination of topical creams, steroid creams, MetroGel, Moritate or Metronidazole along with vitamins, supplements, and natural hormone supplements. Some doctors may find this to be a controversial treatment suggestion.

Maintain clear records of the client's skin type and skin condition.

- Document any reaction to treatments and/or products every time they come in provides you with the best reference tool of your own.

- Determine home care and follow-up salon/spa care.

Set goals for your treatment plan.

- Common goals include decreased redness, tightening of skin, clearer skin, smaller pores, no red or brown spots and smooth moist texture.

- Home Care

  o Cleanser, Toner, Serum, Moisturizer, Sun Protection

  o Antibacterial (Acne), Anti-Aging, Hyperpigmentation, Antioxidants,

  o Eye Serum/Cream, Mask & Lip Mask products

- Follow-up salon/spa care, provide products such as:

  o Cleansers – gel, creamy, cleansing facial bar, medicated ingredients

  o Exfoliants - enzymes (proteolytic), AHA/BHA ingredients (salicylic, glycolic, lactic, azelaic, retinoids)

  o Antibacterial ingredient - benzoyl peroxide

  o Anti-aging ingredients – hyaluronic acid, vitamin C

  o Skin lightening ingredients - hydroquinone, kojic, bilberry, arbutin, mulberry

  o Antioxidants & Free Radical ingredients -Vitamins E, A, & Ester-C

- Mask ingredients for acne - sulfur, clay, bentonite, gel, herbal, self-heating
  - Moisturizer ingredients - hyaluronic, peptides, elastin and collagen, protectant-silicone
- Following up with client
  - Provides you an opportunity to control the products they use.
  - Adjust products with season changes.

TREATMENT PLAN

A treatment plan is the hypothesis and documentation phase. This is where the practitioner/skin therapist records the findings from each skin analysis performed.

- Develop an effective treatment plan.
- Quantify client treatment type (one-time, series or long-term)

DATE: _____

TREATMENT PLAN

1. TODAY'S TREATMENT

- ☐ Skin Analysis
- ☐ Acid Mantle Repair
- Skin Type _____
- ☐ Spa Facial
- ☐ Deep Pore Cleansing
- ☐ Acne

- ☐ Brightening Facial
- ☐ HydraFacial
- ☐ Anti-Aging Facial
- ☐ Rosacea/Sensitive Skin
- ☐ Corrective Program
- ☐ MicroDermabrasion

- ☐ Enzyme _____
- ☐ Peeling Agent _____
- ☐ DermaPlaning
- ☐ MicroNeedling
- ☐ Other _____
  _____

2. TREATMENT DETAILS:

_____
_____
_____
_____
_____

3. TREATMENT PRODUCTS USED:

- ☐ Cleanser _____
- ☐ Exfoliant _____
- ☐ Toner _____
- ☐ Serum _____

- ☐ Massage Oil/Cream _____
- ☐ Moisturizer _____
- ☐ Sunscreen _____
- ☐ Other _____

4. CLIENT FEEDBACK:

_____
_____
_____

5. AFTERCARE/HOMECARE MANAGEMENT:

- ☐ Cleanser _____
- ☐ Toner _____
- ☐ Serum _____
- ☐ Moisturizer _____
- ☐ Sunscreen _____
- ☐ Other _____

NEXT APPOINTMENT: _____

PART TWO

CASE STUDY

CHAPTER 6

SYMONE'S STORY

TCA CHEMICAL PEEL GONE WRONG

This case study is based on a complex treatment using a trichloroacetic acid (TCA) chemical peeling agent that led to unfavorable results. The following synopsis is from the client's interview for the purpose of this book. The intent is to bring to light the ongoing issue in our industry, of liability claims reported for non-reversal facial damage to pigmented skins. This is generally caused by practitioners who are not knowledgeable in the aggressive treatment modalities. In many cases, these treatments should not be applied on pigmented skin or, if an aggressive treatment can be applied, it is mandatory for a pigmented skin to be prepped over a period of time before you begin the application of the aggressive treatment.

The highest percentage of all liability claims in our industry are burns – 28% due to waxing and 21% due to chemical peels. Unfortunately, many practitioners opt to not have insurance.

In the case of Symone, there was no documentation taken, no consent form signed, no prepping of the skin prior to the application of the TCA peel, and no follow-up call. The post peel treatment products given resulted in a fungus infection of her skin. This procedure was showcased on Tik Tok and Instagram without her consent.

I had the opportunity to interview Symone. The following is a photo of her before and after photos.

Note: *The post acne dark spots seen on her before photos are generally found in the upper layers of the epidermis requiring a superficial peeling agent. What she received was a medium depth peel resulting in 2nd degree burns and a fungus infection.*

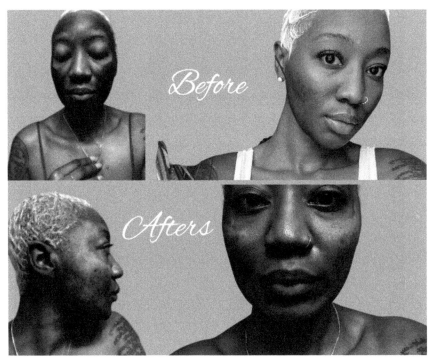

On June 1, 2020, Symone started receiving facial services for hormonal and chemical imbalances due to a severe ICU hospitalization that January. She contracted pneumonia, and acute bronchitis. Since this was during the original inception of COVID, physicians weren't quite sure whether or not she had COVID.

As a result of taking additional medications and steroids, her skin was severely affected. Due to the different medications, she experienced cystic acne and constant breakouts that left post-acne dark spots. She sought the advice of the skin therapist she had been going to for over a year for facials and waxing.

Because of the residual dark spots, the skin therapist recommended a chemical peel. She had been wanting to give Symone a peel previously, but Symone was a flight attendant and her flying schedule did not permit her to stay home for 7-10 days for the peeling process to complete. Symone was aware of the side effects of even doing a light peel; the sun's UV rays, at high altitudes, would cause more damage to her skin.

One year later, Symone began working remotely for the airlines. She reached out to her skin therapist to let her know she was ready to do a chemical peel based on the results of similar treatments she had seen online. Since she was now working at home, it wouldn't be a problem for her to be indoors during the peeling process.

Symone expressed that she wanted to get rid of the post acne dark spots and even out her skin tone. She was charged $150, which included the chemical peel service and a post care kit. The therapist reiterated that she would have to stay indoors since it was summer and very hot outside. When this information was given to her,

Symone stated that she was unaware that the best time for this service was during the cooler months.

The following are questions asked by me, which Symone answered recapping her journey to recover from 2nd degree burns.

When the decision was made to give you a peel -

PAMELA: Did she explain why you needed a peel?

SYMONE: She explained, and I agreed that I needed the peel to help remove the hyperpigmentation spots I had from previous acne and that it (chemical peel) would speed up the process of removing them. The skin therapist advised that a 20% TCA peel was needed because it would be stronger and that doing three layers of it would penetrate better and deeper. She said that TCA peels were better for black skin. She expressed that a previous client she applied the peel to didn't have good results because she didn't peel. So, she believed doing three layers would work on my skin. She also told me that she only trusted me to do this and that she wouldn't do this for anyone else. I know now that because I trusted her, if anything went wrong, she felt I wouldn't react and would be understanding versus if it was done on someone else.

PAMELA: Were you given a "prep" kit to prepare your skin for this deeper peel?

SYMONE: No.

PAMELA: Was a skin analysis performed?

SYMONE: No. She only said, she wanted to dermaplane and microderm the skin so that the peel would penetrate well. I requested that we not dermaplane because I was getting severe cysts/breakouts from it, and she insisted that we do it or the peel wouldn't work.

PAMELA: Did she prepare your skin for the peel with PRO treatments?

SYMONE: No. I went on with my normal skin care routine prior to and on the day of the peel.

PAMELA: How many weeks after the consultation was the peel administered?

SYMONE: That day! She cleansed my face first, then she did microdermabrasion prior to the peel, and she also did dermaplaning. Then she applied the first layer of the TCA peel, and she told me before she applied it that it was going to sting a little bit. I said 'OK.' So, she did the first layer, and it was fine for about three seconds and then from there it was like getting really hot; I could feel the heat coming off my face. She told me, "You know, I'm going to have to do two more layers just because I want it to penetrate really well." And then she said, "just let me know if it gets too painful, but I need to try to keep it on for at least three minutes."

So, she did the second and third layers and it literally felt like my face was on fire. I cannot explain it any other way, outside of the fact that it just felt like the heat was radiating; my eyes were watering, and my body was literally shaking. And then she said, "it's frosting really well… oh… it looks good." And I tried to say, "you've got to make it stop," because it felt like somebody had put a cut on my face and then just poured as much rubbing alcohol as possible on it… and I couldn't take it anymore.

I told her, "You've got to neutralize it, whatever you've got to do… just make it stop!" So, she did, and the heat started to subside a little, but my face was hurting really bad. And mind you, at this point I hadn't seen what my face looked like. She had me lay there for a while… maybe like ten minutes… before she let me see my face. When I had looked up, I saw that she was recording and so she handed me the mirror. She told me, "Before you look at your face, just know it's supposed to be as dark as it is." So, I looked, and it kind of startled me for a bit because from what I saw on the Internet, your face is just supposed to look normal.

I said, "this is really dark!" And she told me, "It's fine, I promise you. You're going to feel so good." And I said OK. But just with me having a little bit of common sense, I told her, "This really looks like a burn, just because I've had my skin burned before and it happened very quickly with it turning into that scab-like material. She then put sunscreen on me, and she also put a homemade concoction on my face … I think it was like peppermint oil, which was going to help penetrate more.

PAMELA: After the application of the peel did you get instructions for your post care?

56

SYMONE: Yes. She didn't want me to cleanse my face for an entire week and she said, "you know, I don't want you to wash your face; I only want you to use the home care kit that I gave you," which was the spray sunscreen and the at-home oil concoction that she made, which she said was going to penetrate more.

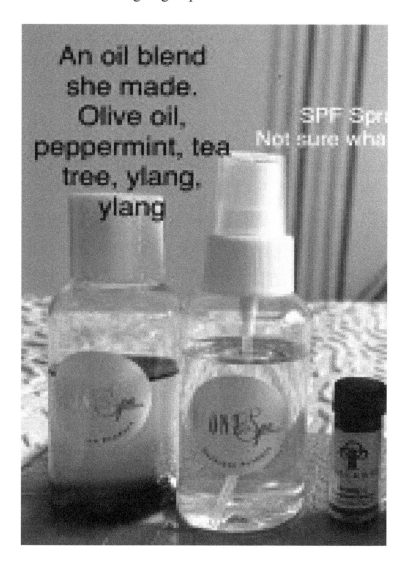

PAMELA: Did you sign any release forms?

SYMONE: No.

PAMELA: Did she call 24 to 48 hours after the peel?

SYMONE: No. I reached out to her when I got home to ask what peel percentage she used, and she stated TCA 20%. She sent me a text on June 13th around 9am saying "Hey Fav. How we feelin' this morning?" I responded with "Hey! I'm feeling good! No pain or sensation. Skin is turning brown and tightening. Just trying to get used to my face looking like this, lol!"

PAMELA: When did you go to a dermatologist?

SYMONE: After seeing a dermatologist on June 22, 2022, she advised me that I couldn't go outside for two months, due to the severity of the post inflammatory hyperpigmentation. Regardless of whether or not I was using SPF, the UV rays during that time would make my face worse and prolong the healing. I was also diagnosed with seborrheic dermatitis and a fungal infection due to the skin therapist's homemade products that were feeding the fungi on my face. I was provided an antifungal medication for the infection and Elidel for the dermatitis. The seborrheic dermatitis was chronic, so I use the Elidel any time I get flare ups from stress, which is my current trigger. The dermatologist also prescribed a compounded skin cream that consisted of a low dose of hydroquinone and tretinoin to speed up the healing of the hyper-pigmentation.

PAMELA: Did this affect your job and pay?

SYMONE: Not so much since I worked remotely but I was unable to do any video calls with my colleagues or clients. I had to keep my camera off for every meeting.

PAMELA: Did you ask for a refund?

SYMONE: Yes, I asked her, via text on June 17th, "Are you able to provide me a refund, please? If not, all is well, and you continue to take care of yourself." She refused to do so.

Peel Instructions

The peel instructions stated, "Peel is not recommended for darker skin tones due to increased risk of post inflammatory hyperpigmentation."

10:34
◀ Messages

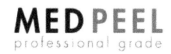

MED PEEL
professional grade

DESCRIPTION   USAGE & INGREDIENTS

WHAT IT IS:

Trichloroacetic Acid, also known as TCA, is an effective chemical agent used to exfoliate and renew skin. TCA can be used to exclusively peel isolated areas of the skin. It is important to note that with applying the 20% TCA peel, it is highly recommended to first begin building up the skin's tolerance by using the **TCA 10% Peel** first with good result. The TCA 20% Peel is not recommended for darker skin tones due to increased risk of post-inflammatory hyperpigmentation.

WHAT IT IS FORMULATED TO DO:

TCA is a deeper penetrating peel than AHA or BHA peels as it exfoliates the skin more rapidly upon initial contact. TC

Symone's Peel Journey

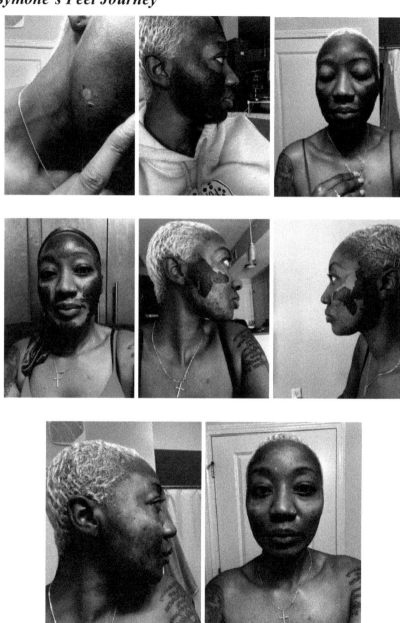

CHAPTER 7

SKIN CONDITION

It Is Important to Know How to Determine Skin Conditions' Primary and Secondary Causes!

Once you understand what the primary and secondary cause is, you can proceed in knowing what treatment modalities address those concerns. In Symone's case, she was concerned about the post acne dark spots, which are superficial post hyperpigmentation lesions.

Primary Cause: Since there is no documentation, the primary cause could not be determined. (Possibilities: oily skin, medication, food intolerance, etc.)

Secondary Cause: Acne breakouts

- Acne must be controlled before removing the dark spots or contemplating on giving a chemical peel. If one is given, it should address the acne, such as a Salicylic or Modified Jessner's solution.

- Home care management products would include low dose of hydroquinone (2%) to be used in the evenings on the affected areas only. AM & PM regimens should include products recommended to control the acne breakouts.

Once under control, address the post acne dark spots (post inflammatory hyperpigmentation).

Before we discuss hyperpigmentation, I want to address the seborrheic dermatitis flareups that Simone is battling.

Seborrheic Dermatitis

After a peel, the skin can be more susceptible to infection. Within a few days to weeks, a bacterial infection can occur. Symone contracted a common chronic and relapsing skin disorder, seborrheic dermatitis, which was caused by a yeast infection.

Seborrheic dermatitis affects the oil glands and causes scaly patches that can present on the face, scalp and other parts of the body. The oil glands in these areas are numerous. The major symptoms are itchy white flakes (dandruff) on the scalp, red or hypopigmented scales on the skin and in infants, a crusty yellow scale called cradle cap.

In some cases, seborrheic dermatitis can be brought on by milia which can appear after a peel. These are tiny white or yellowish bumps that appear on the skin and look like a mild breakout. It is generally part of the healing process. This condition, seborrheic dermatitis, is out of our scope of practice and should be referred to a dermatologist.

Symone is currently seeing a dermatologist who has prescribed Doxycycline for control of her acne. She is still battling with hyperpigmentation and the dermatologist has her on six weeks of hydroquinone, tretinoin and hydrocortisone. For her flareups, she was prescribed Elidel cream.

As a result of the severity of Symone's 2nd degree burn, she has experienced a second type of hyperpigmentation. The second occurrence was from receiving a TCA peel that included dermaplaning, microdermabrasion and three layers of TCA 20%. This aggressive treatment caused the peeling agent to go deep within the epidermis and dermis' papillary layers of the skin.

The severity of the second occurrence was due to her skin not being "prepped" for an aggressive treatment. Possibly if her skin was prepared prior to the application of the TCA peel, the outcome may have not been so severe.

Hyperpigmentation

Hyperpigmentation is the #1 skin condition in melanin-rich skin.

Hyperpigmentation disorders are characterized by the darkening of skin areas due to increased melanin. This may manifest as localized, circumscribed, or diffused lesions of the skin. This group of disorders is frequently observed and may manifest in different forms. In certain parts of the world, hyperpigmentation disorders can be so frequent that they can be in the top list of the most commonly presenting disorders in dermatological clinics.

As recognized, there are two different mechanisms that lead to increased pigmentation. Each of these mechanisms may arise from the epidermis, dermis or from both layers of the skin. Regardless of the area of origin, almost all clients or patients endure the same consequences. As these skin lesions are visible in nature, they can have cosmetic and psychological effects on affected patients. Certain hyperpigmentation conditions lead to long-term disfiguring facial lesions which may affect a person's emotional well-being, social functioning, productivity at work or school, and even self-esteem. What is generally observed in these patients is a reduction in quality of life.

Post inflammatory hyperpigmentation (PIH) is one of the three most commonly presenting hyperpigmentation disorders, followed by freckles and melasma.

When discussing the presentation, causes, and treatment of (PIH), it is important to understand the underlying mechanism of this condition so that we can identify and choose the best protocol for the existing lesions. Even though 'hyperpigmentation disorders' is an umbrella term used to categorize several conditions, each disorder has its own mechanism of origin, which then defines the specific clinical presentations inherited by each condition.

The term 'hyperpigmentation' explains the presence of increased amounts of melanin in the skin by two main mechanisms. Certain hyperpigmentation conditions are caused due to increased melanin production with a normal number of melanocytes in the skin (melanotic hyperpigmentation – post acne dark spots). But there are certain conditions in which the number of melanocytes is increased (melanocytotic hyperpigmentation – 2nd degree burns), leading to an increased melanin production.

Usually, the basal layer (stratum germinativum) of the epidermis contains melanocytes and an increased activity of these cells leads to increased melanin production, which will cause epidermal hyperpigmentation. This is the most commonly found form of hyperpigmentation disorders. In dermal hyperpigmentation, a transferring of epidermally produced melanin to the dermal layer or presence of dermal melanocytes can be observed. Sometimes, a combination of both these mechanisms of melanin production may take place, resulting in mixed hyperpigmentation.

The visible color of hyperpigmentation also depends on the location of the increased melanin production and melanin deposition. An epidermal hyperpigmentation manifests as a brown color lesion and is the most commonly found hyperpigmented lesions. Dermal hyperpigmentation causes blue-gray skin lesions while mixed epidermal hyperpigmentation may result in the formation of brown-gray skin lesions.

Examples of epidermal lesions are ephelides (freckles) and trauma induced lesions (post-inflammatory hyperpigmentation), such as insect bites, post acne dark spots, scratching (dry skin, eczema, etc.).

Dermal melanotic changes can be caused by drugs, a skin condition like melasma, or a disease, and can also result in epidermal and dermal involvement.

The main focus in managing these clients/patients should include identifying the underlying mechanism and cause, and also it is essential to record these patients' histories and progress so that this information will support in optimizing the treatment regimens in the future.

Hyperpigmentation is usually a result of a wide variety of reasons; and sometimes, there is more than one-factor that induces the development of this condition. For the purpose of this book, we will only discuss hyperpigmentation as it relates to post acne dark spots and 2nd degree burns.

Post- Inflammatory Hyperpigmentation

Darker skins are more prone to hyperpigmentation. It is often more intense and lasts longer on darker skin tones. These skin tones are naturally more susceptible to dark spots. The skin is already creating melanin. When trauma is the trigger, it causes the melanocytes (pigment cells) to increase melanin production. Unfortunately, it is more difficult to treat dark spots. The secret is to begin with a conservative approach to ensure the skin does not become irritated or inflamed. Any trauma to a higher Fitzpatrick will cause post-inflammatory hyperpigmentation.

Post-inflammatory type of hyperpigmentation usually occurs after the eruptions of acne and other inflammatory disorders. The post-inflammatory reaction induces melanocytes to assist in the healing of trauma or any inflammatory occurrence.

In Symone's case, the post acne dark spots and 2nd degree burns were caused by

- The inflammatory response from the acne breakouts and,

- mechanically removing the protective barrier by implementing dermaplaning and microdermabrasion procedures as part of the treatment protocol.

However, the trauma and the burn injury have caused her skin to be more prone to UV radiation damage. Wearing sunscreen will prevent the UV rays from stimulating the production of melanin. Therefore, the hyperpigmented areas will not become darker.

The areas of the post acne dark spots and PIH caused by the 2nd degree burn were located in different layers of the skin. The post acne dark spots stimulated increased melanin production in the epidermal layers. The pigmentation increased by the 2nd degree burn led to release of melanin pigment into the papillary part of the dermal layers.

Before choosing a chemical peel, it is important to identify where the PIH is located. A Wood's lamp or skin scope are tools that can distinguish the location of the PIH. Epidermal lesions are seen as light to dark brown lesions on the surface of the skin. Epidermal lesions, under a Wood's lamp or Skin Scope are fluorescent in appearance. It may take up to a year for these lesions to fade on their own.

With the use of tyrosinase inhibitors included in their home care regime and administering pro treatments, fading will be seen in 6 to 12 weeks. Clients must be compliant with the use of home care skin lightening products and broad-spectrum sunscreen, and they should be seen at least once a week or twice per month.

The clinical picture is different for dermal PIH. The lesions are a brownish gray in color and even with examination under a Wood's lamp or Skin Scope the PIH will not be seen visually. In many cases, lesions appear fluorescent, which normally indicates it is in the epidermal layers. Don't be fooled, this could be a "mixed" lesion, meaning it may be in the epidermis and dermis. In this case, only lightening of the lesion will occur. The only option for a better result is referring the client to a laser technician who would combine topical tyrosinase inhibitors with a non-ablative fractional laser. Be sure your referral is with a practitioner experienced in working with pigmented skins.

The identification of PIH can be made after taking a thorough history of the person. In addition, the typical clinical picture also helps to state the cause. However, identifying PIH should state whether it is an epidermal PIH or a dermal PIH. In order to further identify the type of PIH, further investigations should be performed. The clinical identification under a wood lamp, or skin scope examinations help to distinguish between epidermal PIH and dermal PIH. The epidermal PIH examination under one of these tools shows more emphasized borders. However, the dermal PIH under wood lamp examination shows less prominent borders which have very poor visibility.

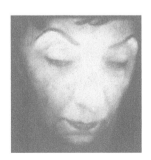

All these tools help to identify very clearly and helps to call out the type of PIH, whether it is epidermal PIH or dermal PIH.

Rx

Generally, the treatment of epidermal PIH is not complex and the treatment needs to be prescribed for a least 6 to 8 treatments. It is easier to treat epidermal PIH than dermal PIH. Epidermal PIH responds well to a conservative treatment, while dermal PIH shows no improvement except for possible use of a non-ablative laser.

One of the important factors that promotes the effectiveness of any treatment is the regular use of broad-spectrum sun protection cream with SPF greater than 15. There are a number of treatment options available; however, most of them show improvement only in the epidermal form of post-inflammatory hyperpigmentation. After a number of trials and errors, it is believed that combination treatment works more effectively than monotherapy.

The application of vitamin serums or cream shows high effectiveness against epidermal PIH. Generally, a greater number of higher Fitzpatricks are affected by PIH. The best combination of treatment for these people is 2% hydroquinone which helps lighten the affected areas. A modified Jessner's solution also is a benefit to use with hydroquinone.

The other topical medication that can be used to treat PIH is Azelaic acid. Azelaic acid works by depigmenting the skin by inhibiting tyrosinase and has the cytotoxic effect on the abnormal melanocytes.

This topical application is highly effective against acne as well as on the PIH caused by acne and other causative factors.

Retinoid is efficacious. Another agent, trichloroacetic acid, in low concentrations of 10% or 20% can be used to diminish the appearance of PIH, which may be in the lower layers of the epidermal layer (melasma) and combine with a tyrosinase inhibitor.

Further, the use of aloe vera leaf extract is believed to be highly efficient in lightening the skin. Aloe vera extract contains a special compound known as aloin, which helps to lighten the skin.

The other familiar product that can be used more efficiently is Kojic Acid, which is usually derived from a certain type of fungus. This acid aids in lightening the skin. However, the efficacy highly depends on the dose; and use of an extremely high amount can cause hyperpigmentation.

The other compound which plays a significant role in PIH treatment is Niacinamide. It is a Vitamin B3, which can prevent the transfer of melanosome to keratinocytes and prevent the melanogenesis. Another vitamin that can also be beneficial in the treatment of PIH is Vitamin C. Vitamin C can stop the tyrosinase activity and also reduces dopaquinone, which is an important compound in melanin production.

The association of PIH is not the primary cause, but the underlying cause of PIH is to blame. The cosmetic defects that are caused by PIH, especially on the crucial locations (cheek, nose, and other facial locations), may lead to serious psychological and emotional stress. In addition, the treatment of epidermal PIH can show a quicker result than dermal PIH.

Management of Hyperpigmentation

The management of hyperpigmentation is usually complex in nature. The management of all types of hyperpigmentation can be divided into two wide groups: conservative therapy and advanced treatment.

The conservative therapy of hyperpigmentation has several topical preparations. The topical preparations are:

- The first line treatment of any hyperpigmentation is with retinoids and hydroquinone 2%. These products are highly efficient in lightening the hyperpigmented region of the skin. However, the treatment with these products needs a longer duration of time to see positive results.

- Azelaic acid is also used in the treatment of hyperpigmentation, especially in the treatment of acne vulgaris induced post-inflammatory hyperpigmentation. The use of Azelaic acid helps to reduce the melanin pigment by inhibiting the tyrosinase. Also, it has a direct cytotoxic effect on the melanocytes, and hence, lightens the skin.

- Kojic acid is a special compound derived from a certain type of fungus, including Aspergillus, penicillium and Acetobacter. This compound also helps to inhibit the activity of tyrosinase, which is the main enzyme needed for the production of melanin pigment from melanocytes.

- Topical retinoids of different generations are effective against hyperpigmentation.

- Glycolic acid peels used as a "carrier" are highly helpful in lightening the skin by applying a skin lightening product, preferably hydroquinone, to the affected areas after neutralizing the acid.

- Trichloroacetic acid is also highly effective in treating the hyperpigmentation and this topical along with cryotherapy is highly useful in Caucasian or fair-skinned people. However, the use of cryotherapy is contraindicated in the dark-skinned people, due to the possible risk of scarring and depigmentation.

- Aloe vera extract that contains aloin, which is a lightening agent, is highly effective against hyperpigmented lesions of all types.

- Niacinamide topical application prevents the transfer of melanosome to keratinocytes and also prevents the melanogenesis. Thus, the depigmentation is achieved.

- As previously mentioned, Vitamin C topical application stops the tyrosinase activity and reduces dopaquinone, which is an important compound in melanin production.

The advanced treatment of hyperpigmentation involves the use of chemical peel layering with the use of actives.

Microdermabrasion – This minimally invasive procedure where the rough skin and uneven layers are removed. This method along with topical application can achieve lightening. This treatment should not be combined with medium-depth peeling agents.

Intense light therapy (pulse light therapy) is also used in the advanced care of hyper-pigmentation for lighter skins, not for darker skin types.

Dermaplaning, microdermabrasion, and TCA peels should not be performed as one treatment, as in Symone's case. It is highly recommended to perform each modality as a separate treatment within 3-to-4-week intervals, due to the risk of hypo or hyperpigmentation.

The reasoning is you will create an uneven surface or epidermis, thus allowing the peel to penetrate unevenly. This will create hot spots and an uncontrollable peel. Depending on the molecular size of the peel solution, it could penetrate to the dermal layer in certain spots more like a fractional laser. Not a desirable outcome when performing facial peels. This will cause crusting, burning, scabbing and scars!

CHAPTER 8

HOME CARE

WHAT TO LOOK FOR IN HOME CARE PRODUCTS FOR DARK SPOTS, DISCOLORATIONS, PATCHES, AND UNEVEN SKIN TONE

In our day-to-day life, we encounter many naturally occurring compounds that have very high efficacy in depigmenting the skin. The naturally occurring products that are scientifically proven in treating hyperpigmentation are:

Artocarpus Communis or breadfruit –The increased intake of this fruit prevents the skin from sunburns due to the presence of a high number of antioxidants and anti-inflammatory agents. The use of breadfruit extract as a topical agent decreases the synthesis of cytosolic phospholipase A_2, cyclooxygenase, nitric oxide synthase and vascular cell adhesion molecules through inhibition of Tumor Necrosis Factor alpha (TNF-Alpha). All these substances are needed to produce sunburn; however, the use of breadfruit topical reduces this substance and hence, prevents the occurrence of sunburn and hyperpigmentation.

Flaxseed oil – Flaxseed oil contains enormous amounts of ALA or Alpha Linolenic Acid. This helps to reduce the hyperpigmentation of the skin. The mechanism by which the ALA depigmenting the skin is not through tyrosinase inhibition, but ALA suppress the synthesis of melanin and accelerates the elimination of melanin from the epidermal layer.

Chia seeds – These small seeds are packed with a very high amount of Linolenic acid. This acid inhibits the melanin production from the alpha cells of melanocytes or melanin alpha cells. This way, chia seed promotes depigmentation of the hyperpigmented area of the skin.

Licorice extract - They contain an active compound called Glabridin. This component has an inhibitory effect on the melanogenesis and also has an inhibitory effect on the tyrosinase.

There are a number of other substances that work by inhibiting the activity of tyrosinase. Tyrosinase is an enzyme which is needed in the melanin production. Hence, this leads to a decline in melanin production and thereby causes a depigmenting effect. The products are:

- Korean based Cyrtomium – this helps in depigmenting the skin by inhibiting the tyrosinase activity and melanin production.
- Ginseng seed extract
- Seaweed – Sargassum polycystium
- Arbutin from bearberry

- Kojic acid from fungus aspergillus, penicillium and acetobacter

- Ellegic acid from cranberry, strawberry, blackberry, walnuts, and grapes

- Aloesin from aloe vera

- Resveratrol from red grapes

- Ox resveratrol from white mulberry

CHAPTER 9

IMPORTANT GUIDELINES

Management of hyperpigmentation disorders can be done by using many aesthetic techniques. But, before coming to a conclusion on how to manage a condition, it is important to understand the complete background of the skin condition. As professionals, it is important to set up a few guidelines so that you will be accurate on your decision, treatment as well as your conclusion while keeping you away from legal issues. Following a set of regular guidelines will help in increasing the standard of the treatments as well as it will improve the conclusion of each condition.

Medical history

Medical history is the most important thing when it comes to a disorder. Every single detail provided by the person who comes to you for treatments is a great help to lead you on the right track. Even though you will meet client/patients with different skin conditions, do not forget that every condition has its own history, and the information the patients provide is always more important than the conclusions you make. Hence, during history taking, try to ask every question that is focused on the complaints the client/patient makes.

Do not forget to ask the onset, progression, associated symptoms and even what exactly bothers them psychologically.

A history of the skin condition is on the first row and should be followed by a family history, which will help you in revealing information if this is related to genetic inheritance or any kind of familial mutations. Also, this will help in revealing any underlying conditions which could be the real cause of the presenting skin condition.

Medications

During history taking it is also important that you ask if the patient was on any kind of medications. This information will help you in knowing possible precipitations of toxic drug reactions that have been manifested as hyperpigmented lesions.

Allergic reactions

Certain medications can cause allergic reactions and make sure you have collected all the information about allergies in the past so that you will not use them in your management protocols. Using allergy-causing drugs can worsen the condition and even, in severe cases, may lead to anaphylactic shock and even cost you your license.

Recording photos of each visit

We all are skin care specialists and for us, the photographs matter as much as the medical records do. That is why, when treating a patient with a skin condition it is important to take photographs of the skin lesions and other visual symptoms during each visit. These photographs should be recorded parallel to the documented summary, which is made during each visit.

There are many advantages in recording photographs. They can help you in catching up all the past details at a single glance. When you go through all the past photos, you will understand if the decision was correct and if the treatment has worked well. The lesions are always better seen than verbally described and that is why many leading skincare clinics do this as a part of their medical guidelines.

Progress tracking

History taking and data recording are performed by all specialists. But progress tracking is a work of a smart professional. Some, clinics and professionals have their own ways of tracking progress. Keeping notes is important. Recording data on charts that record the number of lesions, the size of the lesions or other symptoms over time, would help you make a clear assessment which is specific for each patient. Further, the effectiveness of the treatment can be determined; and if necessary, a dose increment or changing the management regimen can be easily obtained.

Consent forms

Do not forget that even though you are the expert, the client/patient has the sole rights in deciding the treatments. Your client/patient should be the one who chooses it, while you will be only giving options and advice. That is why you have to be always on the safe side. Make sure to get the consent before each treatment modality. A consent form is not necessary during treating a patient with topical

OTC medications. But, during peels, laser therapy, and others, it is necessary to counsel the patient about the procedure and its possible side effects and outcome, and to get the consent. Also, these consent forms should be recorded, as they play a huge role, legally.

CHAPTER 10

SKIN PREPARATION

PRE-PEEL SKIN PREPARATION

The outcome of a chemical service is determined by how the skin was prepped. For darker skin, the concern is manifestation of post treatment hyperpigmentation. Solutions that have deep penetration generate heat while on the skin and/or produces erythema will cause the melanocytes to go into overdrive. When this occurs, excessive melanin is "dropped" at the site of the insult.

Another scenario is the deep penetration causes the melanocyte to be destroyed and no pigment granules can be produced leaving the skin void of color (hypopigmentation).

A Systematic Level of Pre-Treatment.

When it comes to pre-exfoliation or post-treatment, it is important to understand that there are different protocols for each type of treatment and each depth of peel that is performed.

Before getting a chemical peel, some clients need to follow a pre-peel skin care plan for 2 to 4 weeks. This plan can improve results and reduce potential side effects.

Peels range anywhere from lunch time or no downtime peels to some that require a week or more of down time. Having a thorough understanding and knowledge of various types of peels and what falls under the skin care professional's scope of practice is imperative before performing any advanced treatment. Skin care professionals must not only protect themselves, but their clients, as well.

To begin, it is always important to follow the manufacturer's guidelines on the proper use and precautions of the specific peels used. It is also imperative to make sure the specific peels are approved and safe to use on all Fitzpatrick types.

Preparing a client for what their recovery time will be is something that should be discussed ahead of time, as well as frequency of peel and future course of action.

Let's reiterate how the skin receives a chemical peel. Chemical peel solutions generally cause heat when applied to the skin.

- Heat produces erythema. On a lighter skinned individual, the skin is red.
- Erythema is not so readily detected on darker skins.
  - Melanocytes are stimulated, producing excess melanin.
  - Excess melanin creates a concentration of pigment at the site of the insult (post inflammatory hyperpigmentation) or,

o Destroys the melanocyte and skin becomes void of color (post inflammatory hypopigmentation).

The indication for chemical peeling in darker skin is the presence of dyschromias responding to various stimuli, such as:

- Sun

- Medications

- Skin disorders or diseases

The ideal time for giving a chemical peel is during cooler temperatures. Fall, winter and spring are the seasons that have a lower UV index. UV radiation exposure poses varying degrees of risk for all skin types because it has an adverse effect on skin.

PRE-PEEL HOME CARE

The use of "pre-peel" home care products is crucial in minimizing the risk of post inflammatory hyperpigmentation (PIH). The leading cause of PIH is the use of products classified as superficial or medium-depth agents.

All skins should be "prepped" with products that are formulated with an AHA and skin lightening ingredients for a period of 2 to 4 weeks for superficial peels; 4 to 8 weeks for medium depth peels. This pre- peel regimen helps to minimize PIH. In addition, -

- It prepares the skin for a uniform peel.

- Mildly desquamates dead skin cell buildup of the stratum corneum.

- AHAs formulated in a cleanser and toner acts as a "carrier" delivering other product ingredients (such as skin lighteners) into the deeper layers of the skin.

- It decreases melanocyte activity by inhibiting tyrosinase activity preventing PIH.

- Sunscreen compliance is a must to help avoid adverse pigmentary changes.

- Using 2% hydroquinone in the evening for prepping -

  o White to lighter skins allow 2 weeks.

  o Medium to dark skins allow 4 to 6 weeks.

  o Ebony skin tones will require a prepping time of 6 to 8 weeks.

Hydroquinone formulas: over 2 % prepping is reduced to 2 to 4 weeks, depending on the gradient shades of color of the skin.

CHAPTER 11

EXFOLIATION

HOW TO CHOOSE THE CHEMICAL PEELING AGENT THAT MATCHES THE DEPTH OF THE SKIN CONDITION

Progressive, not aggressive, is the golden rule in treating ethnic skin. Once you know where the PIH resides, you can choose the appropriate chemical peeling. If you over treat the issue, meaning you select a chemical peel that addresses a deeper pigment, you may create an unfavorable result. Before going any further let's first, explore the term "exfoliation" of the skin. In some states, the word chemical exfoliation is used instead of chemical peel. The word peel denotes a medical treatment.

Exfoliation

Our skin is in a process of continuous shedding. The skin cells of the epidermis travel from the lower skin layers to the superficial layers. In the most superficial layers, the dead skin cells shed. Depending upon the skin's genetic makeup; at any given time, there are about 15-22 dead skin layers waiting to be sloughed off.

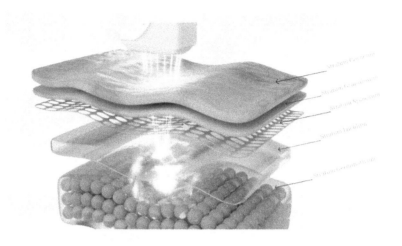

The stratum corneum, which is the most superficial layer of the skin, consists of cells known as corneocytes. The stratum corneum is consistently formed by the process of terminal keratinocyte differentiation. But, in order to maintain a constant thickness of the stratum corneum, it is necessary to shed corneocytes as much as they are being produced. The natural shedding of corneocytes is known as "desquamation". Skin desquamation is the method of physiological skin exfoliation.

The movement of the skin cells from the bottom layers up might not be coordinated and well-regulated all the time. Due to different weather conditions and health problems, the physiological skin exfoliation might get disrupted. The major factors that disrupt physiological skin exfoliation are aging, sun damage and lack of moisture. In these conditions, layers of dead skin will remain accumulated and will give the skin a dull, dry, or damaged look. To restore a healthy glowing skin, it is necessary to use different methods of skin exfoliation and facilitate the shedding of dead skin cells.

Depending on the method used, an aesthetician can determine the depth and strength of exfoliation. The products used to exfoliate the skin are known as "exfoliants" and they can be physical or chemical in nature. The stronger the exfoliant, the deeper it will exfoliate the skin. The deeper the exfoliation, the more the layers of dead skin will be removed. Like in all products, there is a trade-off, even in exfoliants. If you use stronger products and attempt to remove many layers of dead skin at a time, you should be aware that global skins carry a high risk of post inflammatory hyperpigmentation (PIH) and scarring. Therefore, it is necessary to evaluate the ethnic client's skin and formulate a treatment plan based on individual needs and indications.

Types of Exfoliants

Every rubbing, scratching, and wiping off of your skin will remove a few dead cells. These practices cannot remove sufficient amounts of dead cell layers to restore its healthy glow. That is why aestheticians must include exfoliants in their regular skin care regimens and include skin exfoliation in their client's home skin care regimen.

There are two main methods of skin exfoliation, which can provide satisfactory results in skin care:

Physical skin exfoliation

- It mechanically removes the topmost dead skin layers of skin cells. It involves use of scrubs, cleansers, micro beads, loofahs, and sponges that mechanically rub over the skin, removing dead cells adhered to the skin.

Chemical skin exfoliation

- This method uses different chemicals that weaken the bonds between dead skin cells and facilitate their removal.

- It involves chemicals such as Alpha Hydroxy Acids (AHAs), Beta Hydroxy Acids (BHAs), Poly Hydroxy Acids (PHAs) Trichloroacetic Acid and Enzymes.

Physical exfoliants are mostly used routinely for treatment of mild skin conditions that require only a little support to remove the dead skin cells. The scrubs are the most frequently used and can be even applied daily.

On the other hand, chemical peels are used with strict regulations and must be carried out by experts such as dermatologists and aestheticians. The peels and their strengths may vary according to the type and the color of the skin.

The Myth of Hayflick Limit and Exfoliation

Many controversies and discussions were conducted recently on the topic of how exfoliation affects the Hayflick limit of skin cells and affects their turnover. The media circulated many myths causing people to refuse skin exfoliation even in the form of daily scrubbing.

Therefore, it is necessary to understand what Hayflick limit is, and which cells are affected by this physiological function.

Hayflick limit characterizes the number of times a living cell divides before its ability of cell division stops. A cell reaches its Hayflick limit due to shortening of DNA. Shortening of DNA structures called telomeres occurs during every cell cycle and ultimately reaches a level that does not allow the cells to divide further. This happens in around 40-60 cycles.

A lot of skeptics and internet experts have claimed this, regarding human skin cells and made controversies that exfoliation will remove multiple cell layers and will speed up the reach of Hayflick limit in skin cells; and one day, it will cause people to run out of cells to exfoliate.

This is one of the biggest myths! Hayflick limit is applicable only to differentiated cells. But our basement skin cells that produce corneocytes are stem cells. Hayflick limit does not apply to stem cells. Thus, the cells in the basal layer of the epidermis do not have a Hayflick limit. Until the basal layer is intact in a person, corneocytes production will continue. Therefore, there will be skin desquamation as well as need for exfoliation.

On the other hand, the dead skin cells which are removed using exfoliants are already dead cells and they have nothing to do with cell division or Hayflick limit. Thus, by exfoliating, you are facilitating the clients' skin to get rid of unwanted dead skin cells in a coordinated and predictable pattern.

Cell Turnover and Age

Cellular turnover is the speed in which the skin produces new cells and moves from the deepest layers to the top layers of the skin. Slowed cellular turnover is triggered by a decrease in collagen synthesis and elastin (the building blocks of healthy, taut skin), which leads to a loss of skin vibrancy, lift, elasticity, and firmness. The cycle of skin cell production may slow down as we age. It takes about 28 days for a young adult. With advancing age, it may slow down to about 45-60 days or more. When the cell turnover slows down, dead cells accumulate on the surface of the skin causing skin sagging and a collapse of structure, or what we see as lines, wrinkles, and deeper folds. Bacteria can become trapped causing blemishes and breakouts. Skin discolorations and roughness can also be noted. Other factors that affect the skin cycle include hormones, nutrition, sun exposure, illness, and stress.

When the cell turnover is at an average level, the skin looks vibrant and clear with newer cells, and old cells sloughing off. Exfoliation can help in instances where old cells have accumulated.

Integrating Exfoliants in Skincare Routines

It is important to note that exfoliation should be gradually introduced into skincare regimens and should begin with mild exfoliants, such as an enzyme, and move towards stronger exfoliants to facilitate skin adaption.

Indications for Chemical Peeling

The indications for chemical exfoliation depend on the client's desire for correcting skin textural problems. Treatment method, formulations used, and frequency of the procedures may vary with the severity of the condition and the wishes of the client. It is necessary to educate the client about the true outcomes, risks and possible benefits and side effects of procedures before you commence any treatment. Approach each client truthfully, discussing possibilities, risks, benefits, and alternatives.

Here are a few indications for chemical exfoliation:

- Melasma
- Post inflammatory hyperpigmentation
- Freckles
- Lentigines
- Facial melanoses
- Periorbital hyperpigmentation
- Superficial acne scars
- Post acne pigmentation
- Comedonal acne
- Acne vulgaris - Mild to moderately severe acne
- Photoaging
- Fine superficial wrinkling

- Dilated pores (filled with debris accumulation)

- Sunburns

- Milia

- Fine lines and wrinkles

Over-Exfoliation

Skin is not only responsible for your look, but it also carries out several functions. Therefore, it is necessary to maintain the integrity of the skin. Too frequent and aggressive exfoliation may lead to over-exfoliation and skin damage. Although, skin heals well after superficial injuries, frequent damage may cause scarring and pigmentation. Thus, it is necessary to exfoliate the skin, giving it enough time to heal.

Signs of over-exfoliation:

- Skin irritation

- Breakouts

- Burning sensation

- Raw skin

- Ruptured vessels with micro bleeds

The skin renewal cycle is usually twenty-eight days. It is reported that it takes eighty-four days for people over fifty. If you notice any signs of over-exfoliation, make sure you advise the client to avoid exfoliating skin for four weeks continuously. During this period, only use moisturizers and discontinue acid and alcohol-based toners.

Physical Exfoliation	Chemical Exfoliation
Works by mechanically sloughing off the superficial dead skin.	Works by loosening the bonds between dead skin cells in the superficial layers of skin.
Exfoliation is uneven and often can be too abrasive.	Depth of penetration can be determined by the concentration of the chemical peel used and is non-abrasive.
Cannot be used too frequently and vigorously as it may give rise to microinjuries and acne mechanica.	Can be used to treat targeted conditions such as aging, acne, pigmentations, and sunburns.
Avoid rough scrubs when treating sensitive skins (ex, walnut and apricot).	The formulation of the exfoliant can be tailor-made according to skin and needs.
	Avoid recommending high concentration peels at home as they can cause chemical burns and pigmentation.

Physical Exfoliants

Physical exfoliants, also known as scrubs, remove dead skin cells during friction. Scrubs contain small granules that exfoliate dead skin cells on the surface when rubbed on the skin. Physical exfoliants are ideal for the entire body, especially for dry and flaky skin. Scrubs are also beneficial for people with excessively oily skin. Tiny granules cleanse pores and remove dirt, cosmetics, bacteria and roughness, preventing pores from further clogging.

Physical exfoliants most commonly used are:

- Microbeads
- Apricot seeds
- Coffee
- Walnut scrubs
- Sandalwood

If used, these physical exfoliants' warnings should indicate that aggressive pressure may cause post inflammatory hyperpigmentation.

CHAPTER 12

PEELS

CHEMICAL EXFOLIATION (PEELS)

Statistics show there is a high demand for peeling services for Multiethnic patients, but they caution providers to update their knowledge when treating this skin type. Many procedures seem to cause problems for people with dark skin. One of the biggest reasons is that many aestheticians aren't trained to treat dark skin.

Skin conditions appear differently on darker skin. Many conditions are misdiagnosed, which leads to mismanagement and damage to the skin.

The focus of our initial training is more on Caucasian skin types and not on that of people of color. This leads to groups of professionals who have little to no experience providing skincare services for people of color.

Hyperpigmentation and uneven skin tones are a greater concern to the black and brown community. These skins are more susceptible to complications after a chemical peel procedure.

It is best for all new clients or patients, to initially begin a treatment using an enzyme, especially if the barrier is compromised.

Restoration of a healthy barrier generally takes 2 to 3 weeks. Once the barrier is restored to a healthy state, and the pigment is still visible, the skin is prepared to accept more advanced treatments.

Mechanism Of Action of Chemical Peels

Chemical peels are applied to the skin to remove the superficial layers of dead skin cells. It causes removal of several layers of epidermis, and sometimes, dermis, depending on the strength of the exfoliant. It is followed by regeneration of new epidermal and dermal tissues.

The epidermis regenerates from the epidermal appendages, which begins within 24 hours of exfoliation and usually completes within 5-30 days, depending on the age of the individual. The new epidermis that develops after peeling shows better organization and vertical polarity, with a clear and a fresh appearance.

Dermal regeneration is a slower process compared to epidermal regeneration and may take up to several months. The new dermis will have more elasticity and improved organization, with compact horizontally arranged bundles of collagen interspersed with elastic fibers. Telangiectasias or visible blood vessels will be reduced. *Not recommended for global skins.*

Alpha Hydroxy Acids (AHA)

Alpha Hydroxy Acid products are naturally occurring fruit acids and include agents such as -

- Glycolic acid
- Lactic acid
- Mandelic

Alpha-hydroxy acid and other mild acids fall into the category of a superficial peel. They are used to remove only the outer layer of skin and to remove dead skin cells from the most superficial skin layers. Superficial peels are used to improve the quality of skin, remove mild discolorations and rough skin, as well as to refresh the face, neck, chest, or hands.

With Alpha Hydroxy Acids (AHAs), the desquamation begins within a few minutes. The intensity is determined by the pH and the vehicle used. The most widely used AHA is glycolic, which is formulated either with a water base or gel base. The water-based glycolic is known to penetrate more rapidly. The gel-based Glycolic is recommended for higher Fitzpatricks, due to its slower delivery.

As weaker peeling agents, AHAs cause a superficial shock to the cells. They are water-loving or soluble. They create a wound and an inflammatory reaction, thus PIH is a cautionary reaction. Alpha Hydroxy Acids removes bonds between dead cells (desmosomes) and stimulates cell death in deeper layers of the epidermis.

For home care, using a moisturizer with an AHA acid will provide more beneficial effects. These acids act by causing cellular and intercellular swelling and plumping. It leads to an increase in cell and matrix size while reducing the fine lines and discolorations.

Sequential and stepwise treatments will facilitate a smoother complexion and clearer skin. In the case of a sensitive skin that does not respond well to AHA, signs of over-exfoliation may be noted. Skin irritation due to AHA may look similar to the effects caused by retinoid treatment, increased thickness of dermis, increased blood flow to skin and increased sensitivity to sun exposure.

There are three basic types of chemical peels:

- Superficial Peels

- Medium Depth Peels

- Deep Peels

Peeling agent	Histological level of necrosis	Description
Superficial	Stratum corneum to stratum granulosum	Exfoliation of stratum corneum and in higher concentrations can extend to stratum granulosum
Medium	Papillary dermis	Exfoliation of the epidermis and a part of papillary dermis
Deep	Reticular dermis	Exfoliation of the epidermis and papillary dermis extending to reticular dermis

SUPERFICIAL PEELS

Glycolic Acid

Among all the AHAs, the most commonly used in aesthetic treatments is glycolic acid. The other AHAs are combined with different home care product formulations and are used as supportive treatment.

Most aesthetic formulations of skin exfoliation include concentrations of 30% glycolic acid or higher. After a single treatment, subsequent exfoliation takes place for several days. The depth of penetration depends on the amount of time glycolic acid remains on the skin. Therefore, the depth of exfoliation and the subsequent time of its action should be determined before the treatment is carried out.

Many popular AHA home care products contain other acids such as malic acid, lactic acid or glycolic acid in lower concentrations such as 3-10%. These formulations take more time for exfoliation. Such products are sometimes used as a pre-peel primer to potentiate the effects of a higher concentration peel.

Many commercial peeling agents are thickened using glycerin or other mediators. If you prefer using pure AHA gel, make sure it is combined with a thickening agent before applying on the client's skin. This will prevent any liquid running on the skin and will also facilitate equal and even application.

Lactic Acid

Like many other Alpha Hydroxy Acids (AHAs), lactic acid is derived from a food source. In this case, sour milk. It is known to have hydrating properties, modifying the skin surface by promoting skin smoothness. In dry skin, the smoothness is influenced by the recovery of the skin barrier. Other qualities include firming of the epidermal layers, thus softening the appearance of fine lines and wrinkles.

Mandelic Acid

Mandelic acid causes a superficial exfoliation. The penetration is slow and even, due to the larger molecule. It does not stimulate melanosome production which is excellent for higher Fitzpatrick's skin types.

- It is an effective lightening solution for treatment of hyperpigmented lesions.

- Regulates sebum production.

- Provides bacteriostatic action.

Treatment tips if applying an AHA peeling agent -

- Applying a thin layer of the AHA formulation is sufficient as the length of treatment is the major determinant rather than the amount of application.

- Divide the face into 6-8 regions and apply the formulation on each region using a cotton swab, sponge or 2x2 gauze pad.

- Higher concentration of AHA will give the desired result in less time. Therefore, do not leave high concentration formulas for an extended period of time. Exercise caution when using on higher Fitzpatricks.

- Development of a frost is undesirable and indicates deeper depth of destruction. The #1 risk factor for a deeper depth peel is post inflammatory hyperpigmentation for a pigmented skin.

- Applied AHA has to be removed using a neutralizing agent or by cleansing the face with clean water or a neutralizing solution. Always follow the manufacturer's instructions. The neutralizing agents should be based on an alkaline solution such as sodium bicarbonate.

While exfoliation may continue for a few days to weeks, re-epithelialization can be noted within 7-10 days. During that time, the skin is exfoliating after an AHA treatment, and another AHA treatment procedure should not be carried out. If you are using a glycolic series, schedule the next exfoliation treatment 2 to 3 weeks after the previous treatment. Your clients will need multiple AHA treatments to achieve the desired results.

BETA HYDROXY ACIDS (BHA)

While AHAs are water soluble acids made from fruit components, BHAs are fat-soluble and can get deeper into the skin than AHAs. Therefore, BHAs can remove dead skin cells from deep pores and remove excess sebum. It makes BHA the treatment of choice in acne, rosacea, and sunburns. They do not cause a wound or inflammation, rather they denature the protein in the skin. Beta Hydroxy Acids are less likely to cause PIH.

With the help of BHA, an aesthetician can unclog pores, remove the dead skin cells, and remove excess sebum in individuals who suffer from acne. The use of BHAs doesn't make skin sensitive to sun as much as an AHA does. The most common BHA used is - Salicylic.

Medium Depth Peel:

Modified Jessner's solution, Jessner's solutions, Salicylic, and Trichloroacetic acid 20% are considered medium strength peels. They penetrate deeper into dead skin layers, compared to the superficial peels. The treatment is used to improve age spots, fine lines and wrinkles, freckles, and moderate skin discoloration. It also can be used to smooth rough skin and treat some precancerous skin growths, i.e., actinic keratosis.

Salicylic:

Salicylic is a beta hydroxy acid (BHA). It is considered the "healing" agent because of its anti-inflammatory and anti-microbial properties. It functions as a keratolytic agent and enhances the penetration of topical products, such as Vitamins A, C and E, as well as Peptides and oil, and water base products, such as hyaluronic acid. It is the peel of choice for skin types IV to VI proven to show minimal complications in darker skin groups.

Salicylic acid is almost like acetyl salicylic acid (aspirin) and has the same anti-inflammatory properties. The application and use of BHAs are similar to AHA peeling agents.

Jessner's Solutions

Modified Jessner's Solution

The Modified Jessner's solution, also part of the Jessner family, is a non-resorcinol formula with the same equal percentages (14%) of lactic, salicylic, and citric acid ingredients. The citric acid replaces the resorcinol found in the Jessner's solution. Replacing the resorcinol with citric acid allows the penetration of the product to be greatly diminished. This solution works best on sensitive III-VI skin types.

Jessner's Solution

The Jessner's solution is a therapeutic agent that helps to minimize excessive keratinized layers of the stratum corneum prevalent in darker skin types. This solution is considered one of the most effective agents designed for smoothing and addressing the textural pigmentary changes in Skin Types III-VI. It also helps to control acne vulgaris due to its antimicrobial properties while removing lipid buildup that afflicts oily skin. When the excessive lipid buildup is removed, sebaceous follicle debris is easily extracted, and beneficial product ingredients are allowed to penetrate the epidermal layers of the skin.

The most efficacious therapeutic intervention is to understand the various peeling agents and the indication for use. The practical tips given are to reduce risk and enhance results. To lower liability exposure, it is recommended that providers seek professional training prior to administering these solutions on Skin Types III-VI. There is a high incident of post-inflammatory pigmentation and scarring as the major risk factor.

The Jessner's solution is another superficial to medium depth peeling solution depending on the layers applied and is composed of

- 14 g of resorcinol
- 14 g of salicylic acid
- 14 g of lactic acid
- 95% ethanol

These ingredients are mixed to bring the quantity to 100 mL of Jessner's solution.

Application of Modified Jessner's and Jessner's Solutions

These solutions are usually applied with a cotton-tip swab, sponge, or a 2x2 gauze pad. It should be applied evenly to achieve a light but uniform frost. In some cases, multiple coats are applied to achieve the desired results. The frosting achieved with both Jessner's solutions may be accompanied with some side effects, such as feeling heat with a mild discomfort. Some use a fan to control the discomfort of heat.

Personally, I avoid the use of a fan, due to the fact that the solution dries quickly and once it dries, it terminates. After the first layer, the skin generally becomes anesthetized. With the application of additional layers, the discomfort is considerably less.

The special formulations of Jessner's solutions stimulates the skin to initiate its natural peeling, several days after chemical treatment. The superficial epidermis is the target of action; and removal of dead cells and re-generating new epidermal layers can be noted within a few days.

Treatment The client may initially note erythema, dryness, and irritation of the skin.

- This is normal. Some clients may also feel increased skin sensitivity.

- The exfoliation may continue for about a week; and more refreshing and glowing skin can be noted a few days after the treatment.

- The deeper the Jessner peels penetrate the more the time it takes to heal. Stronger peeling agents are phenols.

- Phenols can be used along with various additives such as croton oil and glycerin.

CONTRA-INDICATIONS

- *Anyone Pregnant or Lactating can **Only** receive the Fruit Enzyme Powder Mask

w/Hydrating Complex! DO NOT administer a Glycolic, Salicylic, Modified

Jessner's or Jessner's Solutions!

- *Anyone who has been on Accutane, Retin A, or Isotretinoin, within the past 6-12 months should not receive any peel.

- *Anyone with an active cold sore or fever blister should not receive ANY peel. Refer

client to a physician who will prescribe an antiviral medication such as Acyclovir.

(Zovirax), Famciclovir (Famvir), or Valacyclovir (Valtrex).

- To achieve the best results possible from your peel treatment it is important that you read,

and understand the following instructions.

- If you have any questions regarding these instructions, please contact your skincare

therapist for clarification.

- Please follow the instructions and guidelines provided by your skin therapist.

If for any reason, you stop or interrupt the prep procedure you must contact your skin therapist, immediately. Your scheduled appointment or type of peel may need to be rescheduled.

Ten Days Prior to Your Peel Service Stop/Discontinue These Products and Do Not Have Any of The Following Treatments

* Waxing of any areas to be treated by a peel.

* Depilatory use in any treated area.

* Electrolysis of any treated area.

* Laser/IPL Hair Removal/Photo Rejuvenation treatments of area to be treated by your peel.

* Micro-dermabrasion

* Sun exposure to area to be treated.

* Chemical treatments of any kind including alpha hydroxy acid treatments.

* Hair color/perms or any chemical treatments.

*Notify your skin therapist immediately if you are put on any new type of medication, oral supplement, or any change to your health as it may cause increased sensitivity to your peel treatment.

Procedure Day

On the day of the procedure –

Select an agent by taking into account the percentage and pH of the solution for the best results. It is crucial to understand the agent's percentage and pH as to avoid post treatment hypopigmentation, hyperpigmentation, or scarring.

Initially, lower concentrations should be considered and gradually incorporate higher strengths if the skin will tolerate a higher strength. Superficial agents should range between 2.5 and 3 pH and at a strength of 20 to 30%. The length of time the solution is on the skin should also be taken into account. The clinician should follow the manufacturer's instructions. If performing a series and the manufacturer suggests an agent remain on the skin for up to five minutes, a shorter time frame should be implemented initially for darker skins, i.e., one to two minutes. On subsequent visits, the time may be increased by one-minute increments, if tolerated, until the proposed five minutes is reached. This will prevent excessive burning or creating a "crusting" of the skin. Agents that have the ability to penetrate below the basal layer may cause depigmentation or scarring. The outcome is definitely influenced by the clinician's overall knowledge of the solution's delivery into the skin.

Practical Tips

- Make sure to again explain the steps of the procedure, risks, and outcomes. Remember to have the patient/client sign a consent form prior to administering the procedure.

- Before starting any treatments, take photographs of the clean skin of the face or body, where the treatment will be carried out.

- Provide all the necessary items such as cooling sponges, analgesia (if needed). Make sure you keep all the things ready in the treatment room.

- Carry out the procedure according to the directions and guidelines.

- Take a photograph after the procedure. Taking photographs before and after the procedure should be conducted at each treatment.

- Check the label and expiration date of the peeling agent, as its potency varies with time.

- Take the required quantity of peeling agent in a small glass cup or beaker, inspect for the presence of crystals, and then use the clear fluid. Crystals, if present in the bottle, can adhere to the cotton tip and increase the concentration of the chemical.

- Do not pass the peel bottle or cup over the face of the patient while applying the peel. Keep talking to the patient to allay anxiety, during peel.

- In an apprehensive patient or when trying out a new peel, it is better to do a test peel on the post-auricular area or on a small area on the lesion on the forehead or temple area, instead of a full-face peel.

- Superficial peels carry a lower risk compared to deep peels.

- In high risks clients/patients, different low strength peels can be combined to increase efficacy without increasing risk.

- Chemical peel with a higher pH can also be combined with microdermabrasion to enhance efficacy.

- It is always safe to instruct the client/patient not to schedule an important event or vacation for at least 1-5 days after a superficial peel, and 7-10 days after a medium depth peel.

- Always give your contact number to the client/patient to call if help is needed.

MEDIUM DEPTH POST PEEL HOME CARE

Post exfoliation treatments, the client should be given non-acid products and other home care products. Gentle cleansers, aloe toner, non-acid moisturizer and a broad-spectrum sunscreen must be on the home care list.

For further reassurance, call and check within 24 hours to see if the client is reacting to the treatments and if the client is following home care regimens as indicated. Needed psychological support can also be given over the phone or during treatment sessions.

Instructions for client/patient

Day One

- No water is to be used. Absolutely nothing is to be applied to the skin. The skin should remain untouched. This includes washing hair.

- The skin may have a frosted appearance for a few hours and look sunburned.

- Call your skin therapist if you have any concerns!

Day Two

- The skin starts to turn darker. Do not be alarmed if some areas are darker than others as this is normal. Continue to keep skin dry as in Day One for at least 48 hours post treatment. If skin becomes taut, use a thin layer of Repair Balm or Vaseline.

Day Three

- In the morning, the client is allowed to cleanse the face using an acid-free gentle cleanser. Remind client to be gentle, no rubbing!!

- No-makeup should be worn until after the peeling process is complete.

- The client can use a SPF30 if they must travel outdoors. Wear a hat!

Day Four

- This is the day the peeling process starts. NEVER PEEL OFF SKIN. If long pieces of skin peel, trim them with scissors.

- The skin starts to turn darker and feels much tighter.

- Use a thin layer of Repair Balm or Vaseline to keep skin well-lubricated.

Day Five & Six

- Use same procedure as Day Four.

Day Seven

- The peeling process is normally complete.

- Do not peel or pick off skin since this can cause scarring. Natural peeling will occur throughout this time and will vary with each individual. Client may now begin to use Moisturizer and an SPF30.

Day Eight

- Arrange post peel appointment after the 10th day. Facial should use Gentle Cleanser, Toner without an AHA, Gentle Enzyme; apply a Vitamin C Mask, Gel Mask or Collagen Mask (for Dry Skin).

There are several peeling techniques to use for optimal results:

- Series - weekly or bi-monthly peeling treatments

  o Same peel is given in a series of three to six treatments.

- Combo - combinations of different acids in one solution

  o Modified Jessner's or Jessner's solution.

- Segmental – agents used for combination skin.

  o Combination skin will have the different areas of concern. Give the best peel for each area.

  - Tailored – rotation of different agents (enzyme, lactic acid, salicylic acid, modified Jessner's solution)

TRICHLOROACETIC ACID (TCA)

Trichloroacetic acid (TCA) has been a familiar peeling agent since the early 1980's. The product comes in varying strengths and begins at 2.5% to 50%. There are many skincare companies utilizing low percentages and combination peels. The purchase of TCA's peeling agents is not regulated. Individuals without a current state board license are purchasing the agent through various sources. Preparation of this peeling solution is complex. If done incorrectly, the peel may travel deeper into the layers of the skin than intended, causing irreversible hyperpigmentation or scarring.

INDICATIONS OF TCA PEELING

Listed below are the indications for TCA peeling for skin of color:

Superficial TCA peels	Medium depth TCA peels
Acne	Post-inflammatory hyperpigmentation
Post-inflammatory hyperpigmentation	Superficial acne scars
Epidermal melasma	Keratosis pilaris
Photoaging	Dermal melasma
Dilated pores	Warts
Freckles and lentigines	Lentigines
Rough skin texture	Xanthelasma
Dyschromias	Actinic keratosis
Periorbital melanosis	Seborrheic keratosis

Mechanism of Action of TCA

Trichloroacetic acid acts by coagulating proteins and inducing cell death of the epidermal layer of the skin. This process is known as frosting and the frosting is the end point of peeling. The higher the concentration of the TCA peel, the deeper the layer of skin involved. Coagulation is also followed by inflammation and activation of wound repair, which stimulates new epidermal layer development giving a smoother and even skin tone.

When a skin therapist applies layers of this peel and the frosting becomes a solid white, the solution becomes a medium depth peel. A medium depth peel is a peel that travels to the papillary dermis and should be avoided especially on a person of color. Medium-depth peels have a higher risk of scar formation and must be avoided in Fitzpatrick skin type IV-VI as it may trigger severe post-procedure hyperpigmentation.

TCA is self-neutralizing and thus does not remain in the skin for unwanted lengths of time. It does not enter systemic circulation, making it a safe peel to use in practice. For clients that need superficial improvement, a single application of 10% TCA will be effective.

CAUTION: The number of coats or layers applied will increase the depth of the peel. The more solution is applied, to neutralize itself, it will search for more protein to neutralize itself.

Clients that are prone to post inflammatory hyperpigmentation will need to be pretreated for 4 to 8 weeks with hydroquinone, depending upon the lightness or darkness of the skin. Our scope of practice only allows the use of a 2% hydroquinone.

The percentage of TCA used in medical offices or spas are 5%,10%, and 15%. When used correctly, these percentages will result in the ideal epidermal peel.

Consideration for the depth of the peel:

- Skin Preparation

- Number of coats

- Thickness or wetness of the coats

- The clinician's technique

- Percentage of peel

Peel Depth

TCA falls into the category of moderate-depth peels. The concentrations used in these peels vary from 10% to 50%. Depth of penetration is determined by the concentration and not by the time the solution left on the skin. TCA 50% solution can penetrate deep into the reticular dermis and therefore such concentrations are not recommended as they carry a high risk of damage and scarring. Not recommended for global skins.

In medical spas, a 35% TCA solution is the highest concentration used. The 35% TCA peel has been a traditionally used medium-strength peel. However, when deeper penetration is required, increasing the strength has shown undesirable side effects, such as skin scarring and severe post-procedure inflammation. Research has been conducted on studying the combination of TCA with other agents to improve its depth of penetration while minimizing unwanted skin damage. This strength is not recommended for global skins.

As mentioned previously, for an aesthetician, a TCA 10% to 20% is generally within their scope of practice.

TCA is a keratocoagulant and creates a white frost when it exfoliates the skin. Vigorous rubbing can increase the depth of penetration and thus should be avoided. Some aestheticians use TCA in combination with other peeling agents. For example, Jessner's solution may be applied prior to the application of a 10-20% TCA treatment for a deeper epidermal lesion such as melasma on a global skin type. This practice has shown to produce more uniform penetration of the TCA solution and a more significant outcome.

Treatment tips

- The client's comfort may also be assured by applying sponges soaked in iced saline prior to moving from one facial region to another.

- Sometimes frosting might not appear uniform. If the frosting is not uniform or complete, reapply the solution until frosting of a desired plateau is reached.

TCA treatments will allow the skin to exfoliate for several days. Re-epithelialization will complete within 10-14 days.

You can get variable results depending upon the strengths, patient preparation and application techniques.

All skin types can benefit, however persons with Fitzpatrick IV-VI skin types must be pretreated with hydroquinone to the entire face in the evenings for at least 4 to 8 weeks (depending upon the lightness or darkness of their skin tone) to reduce the incidence of post inflammatory hyperpigmentation.

Frosting

- Level 0– (Full Stratum Corneum) Very Superficial- no frosting or small spots of frost. Skin appears shiny and slick with minimal or no erythema.

- Level 1 (Partial Epidermis) Superficial – frosting is scattered, mild erythema resulting in light flaking. Depth extends into the superficial epidermis.

- Level 2 (Full Epidermis) - Skin has full white frost. Depth extends into the full epidermis with 5 to 7 days of healing.

- Level 3 (Papillary Dermis) - Skin has a uniform solid white color frost, with no skin showing through.

Level 3 frost indicates:

- **Inflammatory Response** - Cell injury
- Injured membranes producing keratinocyte division

Chemical messengers to special cells

- Produces - Undamaged keratinocytes
- Fibroblasts - Resurfacing the wounded area
- Collagen/Elastin - migrating in from the margins of the dermis

- Glucosoaminglycans wound - Process starts within twenty-four hours.

Contraindications for TCA Chemical Peeling

Relative contraindications are determined by the type of the skin of the client, skin sensitivity, and the skin problem that is being treated.

Here are a few absolute contraindications for chemical exfoliation:

- *Active infections*

- *Open wounds*

- *History of drugs with photosensitizing potential*

- *Preexisting inflammatory dermatoses (e.g., psoriasis, atopic dermatitis, pemphigus)*

- *Facial cancers, especially facial melanoma*

- *Uncooperative clients who are careless about sun exposure or application of medicine.*

- *Clients with unrealistic expectations*

- *For medium-depth and deep peels,*
    - history of abnormal scarring, keloids, atrophic skin, or isotretinoin use in the last 12 months

- *Severe sun damage of skin*

- *Previous allergies to any peeling agents and over-reactive skin.*

- *Retin A™, Tazorac or Accutane (all derived from Vitamin A)*

    o Should not be used in conjunction with AHA products or treatments while taking this medication.

- *Salicylic or Jessner's s solutions*

    o Should not be considered if allergic to aspirin.

- Individuals having a history of human immunodeficiency virus (HIV), smoking, or cancer are not good candidates for medium or deep depth peels.

- *Accutane Therapy*

    o If there is a history of Accutane use, application of a chemical solution should not be performed until this therapy is discontinued for six months for superficial peels and twelve months for a medium-deep agent. There is evidence that Accutane may induce an uncontrollable healing response and atypical scarring.

- *Smokers*

    o Heavy smokers are prone to poor healing and are not recommended for medium/deep peels.

- *Sun Exposure*

    o Another variable to consider is UV exposure. Individuals, who work or play excessively in the sun, are not good candidates for chemical procedures.

- o   Insufficient sun protection

- *Herpes Simplex (cold sores)*

  - o   Prophylactic therapy should be administered prior to treatment to prevent an outbreak of cold sores.

- *Diabetes*

  - o   The presence of a disease such as diabetes decreases circulations resulting in wound healing complications.

- *Medications*

  - o   Medications may produce side effects. It is important to know what oral or topical medications the candidate is taking. Refer to a PDR for any contraindications for the medication(s) prescribed.

- *Photosensitizing Drugs*

  - o   Certain prescriptive drugs can sensitize the skin causing dark spots when exposed to UV rays including fixed drug eruptions, which causes dark spots without sun exposure. The most common drugs that are photosensitizing are: some non-steroidals, antihypertensive medications, oral antidiabetic agents, antibiotics, antihistamines, anticonvulsants, hormonal substances, topical antibacterial agents and retinoids.

- *Photosensitizing Essential Oils and Herb*
    - Oil of bergamot, cedar, citron, lavender, lime oil, St. John's Wort, Balsam of Peru (base of perfume) and cologne water.

- *Unrealistic expectations of the client*

What You Should Know

- Not every darker skin has blotchy skin or has dark spots that will be resolved with a chemical exfoliation.

- Most superficial agents do a good job of improving the textural disorders of darker skin.

- Eliminating more serious lesions such as melasma or post inflammatory hyperpigmentation may require a light to medium depth exfoliant.

- Peel concentration of a peel solution percentage (30%) denotes the amount of peeling agent. The pH of 1 to 3 denotes the strength. The lower the pH, the deeper the penetration.

- Necessary supportive home care guidance should all be discussed.

- Consent for the treatments as well as the consent for following post treatment guidelines signed the day of the peel.

- If client is unsure of the treatment, make sure you give some time, reschedule if necessary.

- Do not rush a client to get any treatment or force or convince.

- Layout the real outcomes, possible management methods and risks and let the client decide on their own.

The following is a list of treatments to avoid at least one week prior to a chemical peel:

- Scrubs

- Microdermabrasion

- Depilatories

- Waxing

- Bleaching

- Hair removal lasers

- Threading

- Topical retinoids (avoid 5-7 days prior)

- Any strong skin products

PART THREE

SKIN BURNS

CHAPTER 13

COMPLICATIONS

Chemical peeling is a simple, safe, and cost-effective office procedure. Though complications can occur with peels, they are quite unlikely in well-trained hands. Thorough knowledge about chemical peeling and the risks involved, adequate client/patient counseling and education, and performing peels with all basic precautions minimize the complications of chemical peels.

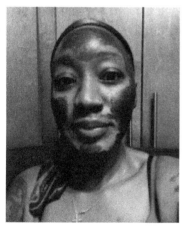

An aesthetician may choose the peeling agent depending on the desired depth of penetration and risks. Exfoliating the epidermis results in rapid healing without scarring is safe. A deeper exfoliation, extending into the papillary or even at times, to reticular dermis, is risky. When using peeling agents that reach the papillary or reticular dermis, the healing is slower, and scarring is most likely for those with pigmented skin. If PIH has reached the papillary or reticular layer, the client should seek the advice of a laser technician who is well-trained in non-ablative laser treatments for skin of color.

Symone's peeling process after the application of two mechanical exfoliations (dermaplaning and microdermabrasion) and a physical

exfoliation (3 layers of TCA). She was diagnosed with 2nd degree burns.

There are many possible complications that may be encountered if you are not knowledgeable with peeling agents. The propensity for complications on diverse ethnic skin is when the skin is not prepped with the proper home care products and/or PRO treatments modalities. Symone experienced many complications that were not adequately addressed.

SKIN BURN

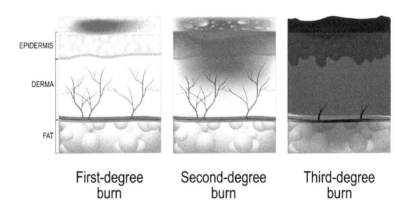

REGENERATIVE MEDICINE IS INFLUENCING THE SKINCARE INDUSTRY

Regenerative medicine includes treatments like exosome therapy which helps to accelerate wound healing after aesthetics procedures.

Exosome Therapy

Exosomes are powerful elements that can restore cells throughout your body. They enhance cell-to-cell communication, which is essential for overall cell health.

Compared to adult stem cells, exosomes contain nearly three times the amount of growth factors. More growth factors mean a better ability to restore and revitalize target cells.

What are exosomes?

Exosomes are nanoparticles released by nearly all cells in the human body, and skin cells have their very own kind of exosomes. They contain various lipids, proteins, amino acids, peptides, growth factors, and genetic material. "They work by communicating and transmitting signals between cells." In the process, exosome therapy increases collagen and elastin production, improves wound healing, and decreases pigment production.

Unfortunately, Symone's 2nd degree burns were not the only complication. She acquired a fungus, which is treatable but not curable.

THE EXPERTISE TO MANAGE THE COMPLICATIONS OF PEELS

In the case of managing a chemical peel, it is defined by the strength of the solution that is applied to the skin. It causes a controlled destruction of the layers of the skin, and is followed by regeneration and remodeling, with improvement of texture and surface abnormality. Though the procedure is generally safe, complications may occur. The various complications that can occur in chemical peeling are:

Immediate (Within minutes to hours after peeling):

- Pruritus, burning, irritation
- Persistent erythema, and edema

Ocular complications delayed (Within a few days to weeks):

- Loss of cutaneous barrier and tissue injury: Infections (bacterial, herpetic, candida)
- Abnormal wound healing: Scarring, delayed healing, milia and textural changes
- Pigmentary changes: Hyperpigmentation, hypopigmentation, demarcation lines
- Adverse reaction to chemical agent: Acneiform eruptions, allergic reactions, toxicity

Though minor, all these complications are more common in darker skin patients and with medium and deep peels as compared to superficial peels.

These complications of chemical peels can be prevented by proper patient selection, patient counseling, adequate priming and with good intra-peel and post-peel care. This chapter outlines some tips to achieve optimal results after chemical peels.

Irritation, Burning, Pruritus, And Pain

The most common complications associated with chemical peeling are described below:

Irritation, burning of the peeled skin, pruritus, and pain are the most common problems associated with chemical peels burns. As we know, chemicals are mainly prepared by acids, which are major causes of these problems. Always keep in mind that these are mild complications associated with skin peeling. Usually burning mostly occurs in the first few hours, irritation in the first few days, and then pruritus and pain.

Prolonged sun exposure, inadequate application of sunscreen, using topical retinoid or glycolic acid immediately after peels can lead to this complication. Paradoxically, in some clients/patients, sunscreens can themselves cause contact sensitization or irritant dermatitis. Pain and burning are commonly encountered during a peel procedure in sensitive skin. It can persist up to 2-5 days after the peel until re-epithelialization is completed.

- Immediate ice application reduces the pain and burning sensation.

- Topical calamine lotion soothes the skin.

- Topical steroids such as hydrocortisone or fluticasone reduce the inflammation.

- Emollients to moisturize the skin.

- Sunscreens to prevent PIH.

Pruritus is defined as itchy skin and can be a normal reaction during the healing process. Hydrocortisone is commonly used. Pruritus is more prevalent after superficial and deep peels, but it can also develop after re-epithelialization. If prolonged pruritus continues, it might be related to contact dermatitis caused by a topical substance (retinoid). If papules, pustules, and erythema appear alongside pruritus, contact dermatitis is likely, and therapy should begin as soon as possible to prevent PIH. It is critical not to begin any additional topical agents during the maintenance phase following the peel. Having erythema with pruritus, burning, or stinging, it is important to rule out current infection or flare-up of a skin disease. This would be the time to seek the diagnosis from a dermatologist.

Pruritus and chronic pruritus disorders disproportionately affects black clients/patients. Management of pruritus of special importance in black clients/patients includes low pH skin care products to protect the skin barrier along with emollients to diminish transepidermal water loss. Further mechanistic studies are needed to characterize racial differences in biomarkers and therapeutic targets of chronic itch. These conditions are easily recognized in Caucasian skin types, but not readily identified in darker skin tones.

Persistent Erythema:

Persistent erythema is characterized by the skin remaining erythematous beyond what is normal for an individual peel. Erythema typically fades in 3-5 days in the superficial peel, 15-30 days in the medium peel, and 60-90 days in the deep peel. Erythema that lasts longer than the above-mentioned time frame is unusual and should be taken seriously. It indicates the possibility of scarring.

Causes of Persistent Erythema:

Persistent erythema mostly occurs due to antigenic factors stimulating vasodilation, which is the widening of blood vessels because of the relaxation of the blood vessel's muscular walls. Vasodilation is a mechanism to enhance blood flow to areas of the body that are lacking oxygen and/or nutrients. This indicates that the growth of fibrous tissue, as in wound healing or in certain diseases, is being stimulated for a prolonged period of time. Hence, it can be accompanied by skin thickening and scarring.

The most common causes of persistent erythema are:

- Usage of topical tretinoin just before and after peel
- Isotretinoin administration prior to peel
- Minimal number of alcoholic beverages.
- Contact dermatitis
- Contact sensitization.
- Exacerbation of pre-existing skin disease
- Genetic susceptibility
- Client peeling skin off prematurely, pickers.

Signs and Symptoms:

The most common signs and symptoms associated with persistent erythema after chemical peeling are:

- Circular, red bumps on the soles, palms, arms, face, and legs that grow into circles that may look like targets.

- Itchiness, in some cases

- Painful sores or blisters on the lips, mouth, eyes

    o Red patches with pale rings inside the patch with purple centers and small blisters called target lesions.

Rx:

Immediate steps are important when you observe the signs and symptoms of persistent erythema after chemical peelings in your client. You should have a working relationship with a doctor or NP to send pictures of the client to; if not, a dermatologist who can treat this condition with topical, systemic, or intraregional steroids if thickening is occurring. You can also use pulsed dye laser to treat the vascular factors.

Edema:

Edema is swelling caused by excess fluid trapped in your body's tissues. Edema is more common with medium and deep peels occurring within 24-72 hrs of chemical peeling. In the case of superficial peels, caution should be used when peeling patients with thin, atrophic, dry skin and in the periocular region, as edema might ensue due to deeper penetration.

Sign and symptoms: Swelling and fluid within the swelling is the most common sign of edema after chemical peeling. You can confirm edema by pressing the affected area. When you press, fluid within the area can confirm your observation.

Rx:

In many cases, edema usually subsides without any treatment. However, whenever you feel swelling and fluid within the swelled area, you can apply ice on the affected area. If referred to a sdermatologist a systemic steroid will most likely be a prescription.

Blistering:

It is more common in younger patients with loose periorbital skin, and around the eyes. Deeper peels, especially AHAs, can cause epidermolysis, vesiculation, and blistering, especially in the sensitive areas such as nasolabial fold and perioral area. Higher percentages of TCA and glycolic acid can cause blistering. Sweating excessively after treatment can irritate the skin or cause blistering due to the sweat being unable to escape through the top layer of dead skin.

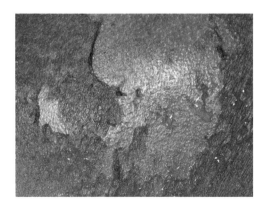

Although TCA is a commonly used peel in lighter skin, trichloroacetic acid (TCA) peel is less frequently preferred in darker skin types, due to the risk of scarring and post-peel dyschromia.

If using a TCA on darker skin, adhere to extreme cautionary measures. The percentage suggested for darker skins is 10%, a lighter skin 20%. Clients should try to avoid sweating until after they have stopped peeling. Therefore, exercise or any activity that causes sweating should be avoided. Avoid picking or lifting the skin prematurely, as this can cause scarring.

The following are conditions that should be treated by a dermatologist. These conditions have been added for the purpose of advanced learning and to identify infectious conditions.

Infections:

Infections are also common complications associated with chemical peeling. Bacterial, fungal, and viral infections are common. Among fungal infection, candida species of the fungus can cause complications after chemical peeling. Similarly, herpes simplex, an important viral infection is common. Bacterial infections may vary, depending upon the type of bacteria affecting the skin. However, E. coli and Pseudomonas are common causes of bacterial infection.

Occurrence of such types of infections depend upon the type of chemical peeling. For example, in case of TCA and phenol peels, there are less chances of infection as these are bactericidal, which means they kill bacteria found on skin. Prolonged application of thick occlusive ointments and poor wound care are the most common predisposing factors of the bacterial infections.

Infections show several clinical features. The most common clinical features are:

- Delayed wound healing

- Folliculitis

- Ulceration, superficial erosions, crusting, and discharge.

Rx: Treatment of the bacterial infection involves several options. One of the best methods to treat the bacterial infection is confirming the organism responsible for infection and then prescribing a drug against this agent. To confirm the presence of a bacterial infection, the physician will swab the area for a culture and sensitivity. Use of topical or oral antibiotic is the best method to treat bacterial infection. Several antibiotic preparations are available for topical use.

Candida Infection:

Candida is the most common species of a fungal infection. Candida infections are quite common after chemical peeling. Superficial pustules can also see in candida infection. Such types of infections are very common after chemical peeling of the immunocompromised patients like in diabetic patients. Oral thrush is another common sign of the candida infection. Oral thrush is characterized by slightly raised, creamy white, sore patches in your mouth or on your tongue.

Rx:

Candida infections after chemical peeling can be treated with use of topical anti-fungal medications prescribed by a dermatologist.

Herpes Infection:

A herpes infection is characterized by reactivation of herpes simplex (a virus) on face and perioral area presenting as sudden appearance of grouped erosions associated with pain. Active herpetic infections can easily be treated with anti-viral agents. A course of Valaciclovir, 1 g twice daily for 10 days may be given. If detected early and treatment is given on time, they do not scar.

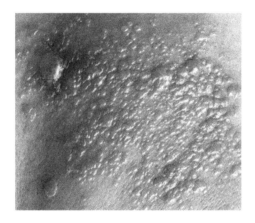

Prevention of herpes simplex: Many patients with a history of herpes simplex should see a physician who may prescribe acyclovir three times a day starting the day of the peel and continuing for 7-14 days, depending on whether the peel is medium or deep. Few advocates acyclovir five times per day or valaciclovir five times per day beginning two days before a peel and continuing for 14 days. Because many patients do not recall earlier herpes simplex infection that occurred years ago, it is preferable to treat all patients with anti-viral medications regardless of a positive history. A negative history of cold sores does not predict the development of post-operative herpes simplex virus infection.

Delayed Healing:

Prolongation of granulation tissue beyond one week to ten days signifies delayed healing. Presence of persistent erythema is a sign of the wound not healing normally. It could be due to the following:

- Infection.
- Contact dermatitis
- Systemic factors

Signs and Symptoms:

Treatment of delayed healing: The best method to treat delayed healing is preventing the bacterial infection. Use all methods that we have discussed in our previous topic to prevent delayed and treat delayed healing. Debridement is another important requirement to treat delayed healing. Treatment of contact allergic or irritant dermatitis with steroids is important. Change of contact agents or protection with a biosynthetic membrane and change dressing along with a close watch on healing skin is a must.

Prevention:

- Strict sun avoidance and use of broad-spectrum sunscreens before and after the peels indefinitely.

- Depigmenting agents (hydroquinone, kojic acid, and arbutin) should be strictly enforced in the post-peel period if residual pigmentation is noted. If there is no resolution of hyperpigmentation after a three-month use of hydroquinone, discontinue.

Milia:

These are inclusion cysts that form during the healing process and are more prevalent with microdermabrasion than with chemical peels. It is most common during the first several weeks of recuperation. Deeper peeling post-peel treatment may promote milia by occluding the higher pilosebaceous units with ointments. Patients with thicker skin are considered to be more vulnerable.

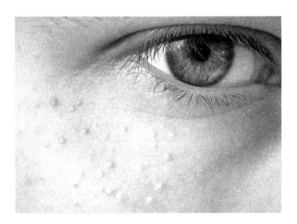

Rx:

Milia frequently resolves spontaneously with routine face cleansing. Extraction or moderate electrodessication (Electrodessication is a quick and simple office-based technique where an electrical current is used to remove specific skin lesions such as sebaceous hyperplasia, cherry angiomas, seborrheic keratoses, skin tags, and brown spots) might be useful in some cases.

Textural changes:

The loss of the stratum corneum might result in the appearance of larger pores post-peel. If the wounding agent is incapable of peeling below the defect, gives an equal depth of wounding, or has a very high surface tension, the selection of this unsuitable wounding agent to peel below defect depth will result in uneven outcomes.

Hyperpigmentation:

It can develop at any moment following a peel and can be chronic if not handled properly. It is the most prevalent side effect of TCA peeling in pigmented skin.

Transient hyperpigmentation or dyschromia are the most common complications of chemical peels, especially in individuals with dark skin. Uneven pigmentation can occur with medium depth peels.

High-risk groups

- Types III-VI skin
- Types I and II skin following intense sun exposure and tanning or use of photo-sensitizing agents.
- Use of photosensitizing agents such as non-steroidal anti-inflammatory drugs, oral contraceptives, etc.
- Early exposure to sunlight without adequate broad-spectrum sunscreens.

- Estrogen containing medication, e.g., oral contraceptives and hormone replacement therapy.

Rx:

To achieve optimum results without side effects, for a superficial peel, the skin should be prepped for approximately two to four weeks depending upon the lightness or darkness of the skin. If the layering technique is going to performed for pigmented lesions in the deeper layers of the skin, skin prepping should occur for four to eight weeks prior to the peel, depending upon the lightness or darkness of the skin. During this time, the skin is being prepped with home care products, and in-clinic PRO treatments should be performed.

- Always perform a patch test, at least 48 hours prior to a chemical peel application.

- In the evenings use a 2% hydroquinone on the affected areas only. If no resolve, in three months, the pigmented lesion most likely resides in the dermis.

- Hydrocortisone cream can be used for several weeks as needed if erythema due to retinoic acid poses a concern.

- Use of broad-spectrum sunscreen with Sun Protection Factor of 30.

Hypopigmentation:

The reversal of hyperpigmentation is hypopigmentation, it's an uncommon adverse effect of a chemical peel therapy, especially when a deep depth is administered. This is when the skin 'loses' its color from its natural tone and creates unattractive discoloration. Those with darker complexion have a higher risk level.

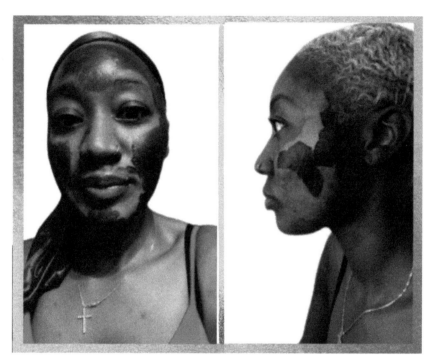

Symone experienced temporary loss of pigment. For those that recover from the loss after a chemical peel, it is due to the peel travelling only through the epidermal layers or to the papillary layers of the skin. When the pigment is restored, the pigment area that was temporarily "void" of color is lighter.

Hypopigmentation occurs when melanin levels in the skin are decreased, resulting in the removal of dark pigment from the skin. This effectively makes the skin more vulnerable to UV rays produced by the sun, as well as making the skin seem blotchy in color. The most prevalent cause of hypopigmentation is skin injury or trauma. Chemical peels have the ability to lighten the skin, while being an uncommon cause of hypopigmentation, because they basically injure the epidermis in order to increase skin cell formation. As with hyperpigmentation, persons with darker skin are more likely to experience undesired skin depigmentation. Deep chemical peels represent the greatest danger of this undesirable skin condition arising.

Prevention:

There are steps to take which can reduce the likelihood of suffering from hypopigmentation.

- It is important you do not administer peeling agents, especially on higher Fitzpatricks, if you are not certified. Certification is important because many consumers look for a certification when seeking these services. The delicacy of the skin requires an apt individual to carry out the steps for a successful outcome. Abalation (removing layers of skin) can produce beautiful or devastating effects; therefore, it is important to choose wisely.

- Clients should not pick the skin when it is in the process of healing. Although it can be tempting to peel the dead layers away to reveal the new skin, this can be seriously damaging and ruin the healing process. Potentially skin could be left scarred and hypopigmented. Be sure to caution clients repeatedly.

- They should follow their post care regimen as instructed.

Allergic Reactions:

Allergic contact dermatitis is more common with resorcinol, salicylic, kojic, lactic acids, and hydroquinone.

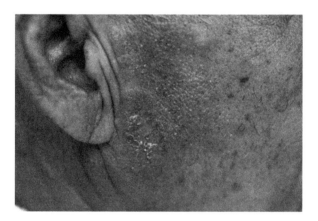

Irritant contact dermatitis can be caused by glycolic acid. Any peel can cause irritant dermatitis when used with excessive frequency, inappropriate high concentration, and vigorous skin preparation using acetone or another degreasing solution.

Predisposing factors

- Beginning a regimen with tretinoin
- Facial shaving
- Use of exfoliating scrubs.

It is important to prepare the skin for a chemical peel. With the use of products that contain ingredients that will remove excess dead layers of the skin. If the client is a higher Fitzpatrick, it is important to apply hydroquinone, a tyrosinase inhibitor. to the entire face for 2 to 8 weeks depending upon the skin tone of the skin.

- The lighter the skin, the average prepping time is 2 to 3 weeks.

- Medium brown skin tones should "prep" for 4 to 5 weeks.

- Darker skin tones should "prep" for 6 to 8 weeks.

- Also, take in consideration the skin condition, the chemical peel being administered and the peel strength (very superficial, superficial, or medium depth)

Additional Precautions

- Closely examine the condition of skin to determine the selection of a chemical peeling agent.

- Elicit if anything has changed since the last intake form was submitted. If so, document those changes.

- If changes occurred, is the client a good chemical peel candidate?

- Did the client/patient "prep" the skin for time needed to lower risk factors?

- Has the client received adequate pre-PRO treatments before administering a chemical peel?

- If the client has herpes simplex, have they received antiviral medication to use as directed?

- Post-peel care instructions explained and given?

- Explain the need for sun protection compliance.

- Beware of habitual skin pickers.

- Beware of those who have a tendency for PIH.

Toxicity:

Instruct clients/patients to notify their practitioner if they have:

- Fever

- Syncopal hypotension (fainting)

- Vomiting, or diarrhea 2-3 days after a peel, followed by a scarlatiniform rash (define) and desquamation.

Other symptoms include:

- Myalgias

- mucosal hyperemia,

Prevention:

- Select only skin types I and II for deep peels.

NOTE: IMMEDIATELY REFER THE FOLLOWING TO A DERMATOLOGIST

Complications	Causes	Prevention
Immediate Pruritus, burning irritation	Dry and sensitive skin Higher concentration of chemical agent	Using calamine lotion in a moisturizing base after the peel. Choosing the right concentration of peeling agent
Persistent erythema and edema.	History of photosensitivity, on photosensitizing drugs, outside occupation.	Proper screening of patients for predisposing factors. Use of broad-spectrum sunscreen with appropriate sun protection factor (SPF)
Ocular complications	Accidental spillage of chemical agent into the eyes	Care should be taken not to pass the bottle over the face of the patient; nner canthus of eye should be protected with petroleum jelly.
Delayed Infections (bacterial, candida, herpetic)	Past history of herpes; picking, scratching, scrubbing the skin can predispose the secondary infections;	Prophylactic antiviral therapy: Use of antibiotics as soon as the warning signs of infection like crusts, oozing, pustules, or blisters

	Inadequate photoprotection. History of keloids or poor wound healing.	appear. Treatment with topical antibiotics and potent topical steroids should be initiated as soon as the early warning signs of scarring like persistent redness, delayed wound healing, infection appear
Scarring, delayed healing, textural changes.		
Hyperpigmentation/hypopigmentation Lines of demarcation Allergic reaction	Darker skin type; deep peels, Inadequate prepping; Improper use of sunscreen. Medium and deep peels in darker skin type Hypersensitivity in atopic individuals	Adequate prepping; Use of broad spectrum sunscreen with appropriate SPF Feathering the edges using peeling agent of lower concentration to merge with surrounding normal skin Test peel in post-auricular region

RESOURCE: B. Anitha, Prevention of Complications in Chemical Peeling

CHAPTER 14

PATIENT MANAGEMENT

PATIENT SELECTION

The first step in preventing complications is to identify the patients at risk, so that complications can be anticipated, prevented, and if they still happen, treated at the earliest. These patients include those-

- with darker skin types with a tendency to develop post inflammatory hyperpigmentation.

- with sensitive skin or history of atopic dermatitis

- with dry skin and a reddish hue

- with outdoor occupations

- with history of photosensitivity or post inflammatory hyperpigmentation on photosensitizing drugs

- with history of keloids or poor wound healing or herpes infection

- who have recently received isotretinoin with unrealistic expectations, uncooperative and fussy patients and

- who are psychologically disturbed.

PATIENT COUNSELING

A detailed consent form should be taken. Pre-peel photography under proper lighting is advised in all cases. The patient should be specifically counselled about:

- the nature of the treatment,

- the risks involved,

- the expected results,

- the early warning signs like erythema, hyperpigmentation, crusting, etc.,

- the need for applying proper topical treatment after peels for maintenance and preventing complications and

- the need for avoidance of sun, irritant chemicals, etc.

PRE-PEEL PRECAUTIONS

The pre-peel precautions to be taken to prevent complications include identifying the patients at risk by a detailed history and examination as specified above. Other precautions include the following.

- Adequate prepping of the skin for at least 2-4 weeks prior to peel and discontinuing 3-5 days before the procedure is of vital importance. Priming is done by application of depigmenting agents such as hydroquinone and use of sunscreens.

- Patient should be instructed not to bleach, wax, scrub, massage or use depilatories or scrubs, or schedule any important event 1 week before the peel and to stop retinoid three days before the peel.

- In patients with active lesion or herpes simplex, a prophylactic antiviral such as acyclovir five times a day, or valaciclovir three times a day, should be given, according to the physician's recommendation until re-epithelialization occurs.

PEEL PRECAUTIONS

- While doing a chemical peel, it is very important to select the right peeling agent at the right concentration.

- It is always better to under peel than over peel in the initial stages.

- Sensitive areas like the inner canthus of the eye and nasolabial folds should be protected with petroleum jelly.

- The neutralizing agent must be kept ready to terminate the peel if required before the scheduled time.

- When peeling the periorbital area, a dry swab stick must be kept ready to absorb any tears. If there is watering of the eyes, the peel can trickle up or down.

- When doing medium and deep peels, especially in darker skin, peeling agent with lower concentration should be feathered at the edges to merge with the surrounding normal skin to avoid lines of demarcation.

POST-PEEL CARE

Good post procedure care ensures early recovery with minimal complications.

a. In the immediate post peel period, gentle or non-soap cleanser should be used.

b. If there is crusting, topical antibiotic ointment should be used to prevent bacterial infection and enhance wound healing.

c. Sun exposure should be avoided and broad spectrum sunscreen should be used meticulously.

d. Calamine lotion in a moisturizing base can be used for stinging sensation.

e. Peeling agents like glycolic acid and retinoids should be avoided till desquamation is complete and given consent by the practitioner.

f. Patients should be strictly warned against picking, peeling, scratching, rubbing or scrubbing the skin.

g. Patients should be clearly informed to recognize complications like excessive redness, swelling, burning or pain, crusts, oozing, pus formation or blisters and to report immediately to a dermatologist, so that preventive actions can be taken promptly.

PART FOUR

INSURANCE

CHAPTER 15

LIABILITY INSURANCE

It has been noted that many skin therapists are opting to not have liability insurance to cover them or their business. *Here are the statistics:*

The #1 liability claims are burns with aestheticians who are causing both waxing and chemical peels. Of all claims recorded, 28% from waxing and 21% from chemical peels.

Here is an article provided by the U.S. Small Business Association (SB)

Get Business Insurance

Business insurance protects you from the unexpected costs of running a business. Accidents, natural disasters, and lawsuits could run you out of business if you're not protected with the right insurance.

Pick the type of business insurance you need.

The protections you get from choosing a business structure like a limited liability company (LLC) or a corporation typically only protect your personal property from lawsuits, and even that protection is limited. Business insurance can fill in the gaps to make sure both your personal assets and your business assets are fully protected from unexpected catastrophes. In some instances, you might be legally required to purchase certain types of business insurance. The federal government requires every business with employees to have workers' compensation, unemployment, and disability insurance. Some states also require additional insurance. Laws requiring insurance vary by state, so visit your state's website to find out the requirements for your business.

Six Common Types of Business Insurance

After you purchase insurance that's required by law, you can find insurance to cover any other business risk. As a general rule, you should insure against things you wouldn't be able to pay for on your own. Speak to insurance agents to find out what kinds of coverage makes sense for your business and compare terms and prices to find the best deal for you.

Here are six common kinds of business insurance to look for:

Insurance Type	Who It's For	What It Does
General liability insurance	Any business	This coverage protects against financial loss as the result of bodily injury, property damage, medical expenses, libel, slander, defending lawsuits, and settlement bonds or judgments.

Insurance Type	Who It's For	What It Does
Product liability insurance	Businesses that manufacture, wholesale, distribute, and retail a product	This coverage protects against financial loss as a result of a defective product that causes injury or bodily harm.
Professional liability insurance	Businesses that provide services to customers	This coverage protects against financial loss as a result of malpractice, errors, and negligence.
Commercial property insurance	Businesses with a significant amount of property and physical assets	This coverage protects your business against loss and damage of company property due to a wide variety of events such as fire, smoke, wind and hailstorms, civil disobedience, and vandalism.
Home-based business insurance	Businesses that are run out of the owner's personal home	Coverage that's added to homeowner's insurance as a rider can offer protection for a small amount of business equipment and liability coverage for third-party injuries.
Business owner's policy	Most small business owners, but especially home-based business owners	A business owner's policy is an insurance package that combines all of the typical coverage options into one bundle. They simplify the insurance buying process and can save you money.

Four steps to buy business insurance:

1. **Assess your risks**. Think about what kind of accidents, natural disasters, or lawsuits could damage your business. For example, if your business is located in a commercial area that is at risk from seasonal events such as fire or hail storms, commercial property insurance will help protect against loss.

2. **Find a reputable licensed agent**. Commercial insurance agents can help you find policies that match your business needs. They receive commissions from insurance companies when they sell policies, so it's important to find a licensed agent that is interested in your needs as much as his or her own needs.

3. **Shop around.** Prices and benefits can vary significantly. You should compare rates, terms, and benefits for insurance offers from several different agents.

4. **Re-assess every year**. As your business grows, so do your liabilities. If you have purchased or replaced equipment or expanded operations, you should contact your insurance agent to discuss changes in your business and how they affect your coverage.

What Every Solo Esthetician Should Know About Insurance

In this sue-happy age, it is expensive to defend yourself, even when you've done nothing wrong. Smart independent esties realize that being named in a lawsuit is not worth risking their career. As a solo esthetician, you probably know that you will need insurance, but did you know there are several types of insurance, and you may need different policies for different risks?

The following are blogs provided by Associated Skin Care Professionals (ASCP)

What is Liability Insurance?

First, what exactly is liability insurance? What does it do? Why is it important? It is an insurance policy that protects you when you are being sued and/or being held legally liable for claims of negligence resulting from damage or injury to a person or property.

Simply put, you have been negligent in some way at work, and it resulted in injury to a client or damaged their property in some way.

Here's information on insurance types:

What is Professional Liability?

Professional Liability is when a client has been injured during the service you performed.

- For instance, glass falling out of a mag lamp and cutting the orbital bone on a client or a steamer spitting scalding water and burning a client—accidents happen.

What is Product Liability?

Product Liability is when a client has suffered an allergic reaction caused from a product used on them or sold to them for at-home use.

- An example of this is a rash developing from a client overusing their glycolic acid cleanser.

What is General Liability?

- General Liability is when a client has been injured during a slip and fall, or due to faulty equipment. This also covers damage to a client's property from faulty equipment.

- An example of this is when one of our members traveled to a client's house to perform a facial. After the facial was complete, the member went to pack up her supplies and noticed the products had left permanent rings on an antique wood table, ruining the table. Guess how much the table cost? $10,000! Thankfully, the member had insurance, which covered the price of this costly mistake.

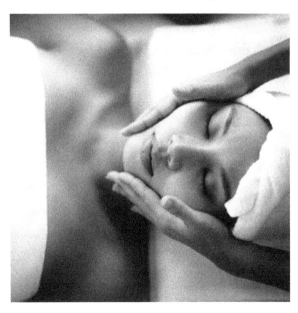

CHAPTER 16

BUSINESS PERSONAL PROPERTY INSURANCE

Business Personal Property (BPP) Insurance is contents coverage for your business. This valuable insurance meets the solo esthetician's needs in the event of equipment loss due to a fire, flood, or theft.

Shared Vs. Individual Coverage

To be sure your insurance coverage is your own and is not shared with other policyholders, make sure the aggregate coverage on your policy is per individual, per year—not a shared master aggregate.

Why does this matter? If you purchase a policy with a shared master aggregate, it means you are sharing the insurance policy limits with fellow policyholders.

Let's say your insurance provider has a particularly high number of claims in one year from their other customers and pays out several sizeable settlements to those people. If you file a claim of your own later in the year, it's possible there may be no money left to defend or settle your claim. With an individual aggregate policy, the policy limits are available to you (and you only) for the entire policy year.

Occurrence Form Vs. Claims-Made

Also ask if the policy is a claims-made policy or an occurrence form policy.

Claims-made coverage requires claims be reported while your policy is in effect. If your policy has expired and someone makes a claim against you (even though you had insurance at the time of the incident), you will have no insurance coverage because your policy has lapsed. The insurance company also has the right to refuse to renew your policy. This could make it difficult to protect yourself.

Occurrence form means coverage continues for incidents that occur while you were insured, even if a claim is filed later when your policy has lapsed. With occurrence form coverage, should you have a claim filed 23 months later, even though you no longer have a current policy, your policy will provide liability coverage for a covered claim.

Esthetician Insurance with ASCP

Smart estheticians realize that being named in a lawsuit is not worth risking your career. In this sue-happy age, it is expensive to defend yourself even when you've done nothing wrong. Why chance it when excellent protection is so affordable?

Associated Skin Care Professionals (ASCP) offers protection with the industry's best value in liability coverage for skin care professionals. For only $259 per year, you receive:

- $2 million per occurrence

- $6 million total per policy year (for YOU, not shared with other professionals)

- Covers professional, general, and product liability

- Covers you wherever you work, no matter how many settings

Not an ASCP Member? Join Today!

Scarred For Life

When Rhonda finally got her dream job at a luxury spa, she never dreamed she would soon be living in fear of losing her house. When Rhonda first became employed at the spa, her manager assured her all the treatments she would be performing were covered under the spa's insurance. Rhonda never thought to confirm this with the spa.

On this day, Rhonda performed an IPL hair removal service as she had always done. During the treatment, the client said she felt heat in a few areas on her leg. Rhonda told the client she would avoid those areas and continue with the treatment. Following the treatment, she gave her client the post-treatment care instructions; the client seemed happy and left.

Several weeks later, Rhonda came home from work to find a court summons taped to the front door of her home. The client was suing Rhonda for $600,000 in damages and medical bills resulting from scarring to 25% of her legs. Unfortunately, the spa had let their coverage lapse and Rhonda was not covered.

The client settled in court for $126,000. Unfortunately, the client was not the only one burned in this case. Rhonda was not an ASCP member.

Employer Coverage

Never assume you are covered by your employer. We have heard some incredibly sad stories of estheticians who relied on their employer's policy and found out too late that they were not covered.

There are four important questions you should ask your employer to ensure you do have complete coverage that protects you as an individual. And remember, your employer's coverage is not going to cover you if you are practicing outside your employer's domain. So, if you if plan to work on family and friends, make sure they are coming to see you at your place of business.

Am I covered if my client sues me INDIVIDUALLY?

An employer's insurance policy protects the business and its owner in the event they are sued. If you are also named by your client in a lawsuit, and the employer's policy does not explicitly provide coverage for you, the individual therapist, you stand a chance of losing your personal assets, such as your house, your car, and/or your savings.

If you plan on being covered under your employer's insurance, take a good look at their policy, and ask some of these follow-up questions:

Does the employer's policy cover every treatment you're performing?

Many traditional insurance companies do not understand esthetics…at least not like ASCP does. Many of them will not cover eyelash extensions. Some don't cover Brazilian waxing. Some will not even cover chemical peels. You might end up doing a service several times a day and not be covered. And this isn't something you want to find out after an incident has occurred. Confirm that all services you perform are included in your employer's policy.

Is the employer's policy current? Do they renew the policy on time?

Bills can get lost in the mail; we can lose track of time . . . a lot can happen. We're human and we're busy people. But if your employer doesn't renew the policy on time and you end up injuring a client during that period lapse, you will not be covered. Obtaining your own policy is the best way to ensure you are covered.

Are you covered everywhere you work?

If you do any work outside that place of business, your employer is not going to cover you. They will only cover you for incidents that happen while you are working under their roof, for them. ASCP membership and insurance will follow you wherever you work, no matter how many settings.

NOTE: This chapter was provided by Associated Skin Care Professionals, visit www.ascpskincare.com for more information

SCAN ME W/CAMERA

Licensed aestheticians, scan the QR code to purchase liability insurance for only $209 – a savings of $50

REFERENCES

http://www.aafp.org/afp/2003/1115/p1955.html

http://www.medscape.com/viewarticle/493946

http://emedicine.medscape.com/article/1069686-overview

http://www.dermnetnz.org/topics/pigmentation-disorders/

http://www.medscape.org/viewarticle/587472

https://www.truthinadvertising.org/wp-content/uploads/2013/10/medscape-hyperpigmentation.pdf

http://www.msdmanuals.com/professional/dermatologic-disorders/pigmentation-disorders/hyperpigmentation

http://www.derm-sinica.com/article/S1027-8117(14)00045-7/abstract

https://www.ncbi.nlm.nih.gov/pmc/articles/PMC2921758/

https://www.ncbi.nlm.nih.gov/pmc/articles/PMC3388446/

https://www.ncbi.nlm.nih.gov/pmc/articles/PMC3938350/

http://onlinelibrary.wiley.com/doi/10.1111/j.1600-0560.1982.tb01069.x/full

Books

Illustrated synopsis of dermatology and sexually transmitted diseases - Neena Khanna

RESOURCES

Prevention of Complications in Chemical Peeling, B Anitha, J Cutan Aesthet Surg. 2010 Sep-Dec; 3(3): 186–188. doi: 10.4103/0974-2077.74500. PMCID: PMC3047741

Khunger N. Step by step chemical peels. 1st ed. New Delhi: Jaypee Medical Publishers; 2009. Complications; pp. 280–97.

Khunger N. Standard guidelines of care for chemical peels. Indian J Dermatol Venereol Leprol. 2008;74:S5–12.

Bari AU, Iqbal Z, Rahman SB. Tolerance and safety of superficial chemical peeling with salicylic acid in various facial dermatoses. Indian J Dermatol Venereol Leprol. 2005;71:87–90.

Resnik SS, Resnik BI. Complications of chemical peeling. Dermatol Clin. 1995;13:309–12.

Briden ME. Alpha-hydroxyacid chemical peeling agents: Case studies and rationale for safe and effective use. Cutis. 2004;73:18–24

Khunger N. Chemical peels. In: Khunger N, Sachdev M, editors. Practical Manual of Cosmetic Dermatology and Surgery. 1st ed. New Delhi, India: Mehta Publishers; 2010. pp. 326–36.

Duffy DM. Avoiding complications with chemical peels. In: Rubin MG, editor. Procedures in cosmetic dermatology series: Chemical peels. Amsterdam: Elsevier Inc; 2006. pp. 137–70.

Fung JF, Sengelmann RD, Kenneally CZ. Chemical injury to the eye from trichloroacetic acid. Dermatol Surg. 2002;28:609–10.

Rendon MI, Berson DS, Cohen JL, Roberts WE, Starker I, Wang B. Evidence and considerations in the application of chemical peels in skin disorders and aesthetic resurfacing. J Clin Aesthetic Dermatol. 2010;3:32–43.

http://journals.lww.com/jdnaonline/Fulltext/2011/07000/Anatomy_and_Physiology_of_the_Skin.3.aspx

http://onlinelibrary.wiley.com/doi/10.1111/j.1524-4725.1997.tb00003.x/full

http://europepmc.org/abstract/med/7600706

http://onlinelibrary.wiley.com/doi/10.1111/j.1524-4725.1996.tb00343.x/full

http://onlinelibrary.wiley.com/doi/10.1111/j.1524-4725.1997.tb00014.x/full

http://www.webmd.com/vitamins-supplements/ingredientmono-977-alpha%20hydroxy%20acids.aspx?activeingredientid=977&activeingredientname=alpha%20hydroxy%20acids

http://www.webmd.com/vitamins-supplements/ingredientmono-977-alpha%20hydroxy%20acids.aspx?activeingredientid=977&activeingredientname=alpha%20hydroxy%20acids

https://www.google.com/patents/US4767750

http://onlinelibrary.wiley.com/doi/10.1046/j.1524-4725.1999.08145.x/full

http://onlinelibrary.wiley.com/doi/10.1111/j.1524-4725.2003.29384.x/full

http://www.dermage.com.br/dermage/paginas/article.pdf

http://onlinelibrary.wiley.com/doi/10.1111/j.1524-4725.2008.34383.x/full

https://www.google.com/patents/US5153230

https://books.google.lk/books?hl=en&lr=&id=JpfgVgb62nsC&oi=fnd&pg=PA213&dq=glycerine+for+dry+skin&ots=flAowWxoCp&sig=hYhZlcoPIfEJQSwoGckblbYKwew&redir_esc=y#v=onepage&q=glycerine%20for%20dry%20skin&f=false

Pruritus in Black Skin: Unique Molecular Characteristics and Clinical Features: Michael McColl, Emily Boozalis, Crystal Aquh, AmarachiC Eseony Ginette A Okaoye, Shawn G Kwatra

ABOUT THE AUTHOR

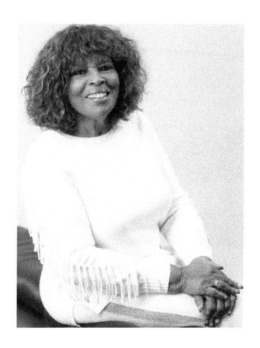

Pamela Springer's aesthetics knowledge has given her recognition as a leader in advanced aesthetics education. She is a highly sought-after professional speaker for TV, medical conferences, and aesthetic trade shows. She has appeared on Oprah, and as a skincare expert on stations, such as Fox, NBC, and ABC stations, nationally.

As a professional speaker, Ms. Springer addresses the beauty industry's lack of specialized training when it comes to the skin differences between people of other races. Her company, Global

Skin Solutions, LLC has become a national continuing education provider for the California Board of Registering Nurses. Being a CE provider allows Springer to train medical staff on the nuances of ethnic skin; how to lower risk factors and enhance results.

Pamela began her career in the beauty industry as a National Training Director for the first major ethnic skincare company. She soon discovered the lack of education in pigmentation and the understanding of diverse ethnic skin. As an African American woman who has a mixed ancestry from three other lineages, her passion became educating other skincare professionals on the unique nuances of ethnic pigmented skin.

Before opening The Skin & Makeup Institute of Arizona in 2000, Pamela completed a 9-month preceptorship under the tutelage of a board-certified dermatologist and medical school professor specializing in Ethno-Dermatology.

Springer launched Global Skin Solutions LLC, a corrective skincare line in 2009. In 2011, Global Skin Solutions (GSS) received a board-certified dermatologist product endorsement and recommendation. GSS is formulated to reflect the unique challenges that professionals face in providing treatment modalities for today's diverse ethnic skincare market.

 Her certification courses are based on Ethno-Dermatology science-related didactics and evidence-based treatment modalities. This certification program provides advanced aesthetics training in understanding the genetic composition; gives answers to therapeutically challenging pigment disorders; and imparts cultural diversity information. Medspas and spas around the country are receiving Certification in Skin of Color to assure their licensed professional are confident to address all diverse skin tones and their skincare needs.

Pamela has also authored, *Don't Be Afraid of the Dark - Learn How to Master Chemical Peels and More...for a world of diverse skin tones.* This book is a valuable resource containing the latest in ethnic skincare. It is based on science yet **presented in a manner that is easy to understand**.

BEST SELLER!

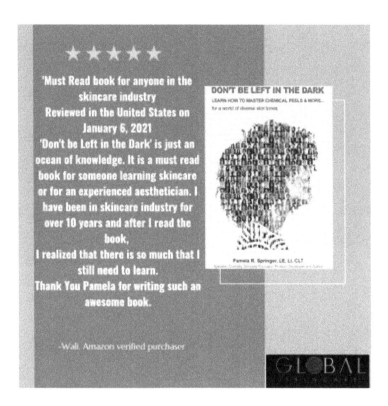

SCAN ME W/CAMERA

Printed in the USA
CPSIA information can be obtained
at www.ICGtesting.com
LVHW051948211123
764224LV00107B/5367